PILLS THAT DON'T WORK

PILLS THAT DON'T WORK

a consumers' and
doctors' guide to
over 600 prescription
drugs that lack
evidence of
effectiveness

by
SIDNEY M. WOLFE, M.D.
CHRISTOPHER M. COLEY
and the
HEALTH
RESEARCH
GROUP,
founded by Ralph Nader

FARRAR STRAUS GIROUX
NEW YORK

Printed in the United States of America
Published simultaneously in Canada by
McGraw-Hill Ryerson Ltd., Toronto

Library of Congress Cataloging in Publication Data
Wolfe, Sidney M. Pills that don't work.
  Bibliography: p.   Includes index.
  1. Drugs—Effectiveness. 2. Drugs—Safety measures.
I. Coley, Christopher M. II. Public Citizen, inc.
Health Research Group. III. Title.
RM301.W64   615'.7   81-5422
ISBN 0-374-23341-1   AACR2
ISBN 0-374-51662-6 (pbk.)

ACKNOWLEDGMENTS

Pills That Don't Work is the result of an extraordinary and rewarding effort by the staff of the Public Citizen Health Research Group with generous help and advice from many others outside the group. All have authored the book.

Health Research Group Staff:

• Phyllis McCarthy and Laurie Pyne not only typed and proofread the manuscript again and again, but edited and made many valuable suggestions which have improved the book.

• Judy Portnoy did the original research on expenditures for ineffective drugs, helped to shape the style of the book and did endless editing and proofreading.

• Mike Behrman helped research several sections of the book and made valuable contributions editing and proofreading.

• Linda Cahill provided the artwork for the cover, oversaw the entire production of the book, coached everyone and made the book happen.

• Lisa Northcutt helped with the distribution and reprinting of the book.

• Eve Bargmann, M.D., Ben Gordon, Rob Leflar, Marcia Goldberg, Pauline Sobel, Al Harris and John Laskey all helped with editing or proofreading, and Dan Sigelman and Henry Bergman encouraged everyone else.

Others

• Margaret Sharkey volunteered a great deal of time and patience typing and editing the original drafts of the manuscripts.

• Judy Harkison contributed valuable editing of the book.

• Vern Allen and Lanny Tupper spent many long hours typesetting, retypesetting and laying out the book.

• Frank O'Brien, Joe Byrne and John Guyton, as well as the many temporary and volunteer workers in the Public Citizen Administration office, spent many hours making sure the book reached the people.

• Bill Schultz and John Sims, staff attorneys from Public Citizen Litigation Group, reviewed the book and contributed valuable advice on its contents.

- Dr. Michael Newman, who practices Internal Medicine in Washington, D.C., Dr. Quentin Young, Chief of Medicine of Cook County Hospital in Chicago, Illinois, and Dr. Samuel Itscoitz, a cardiologist in Washington, D.C., all read the manuscript and made important suggestions which improved the book.

- Dr. Sumner Kalman, a physician and professor of pharmacology at Stanford University School of Medicine, reviewed the manuscript and had many helpful comments which we incorporated into the book.

- Dr. Paul Stolley, professor of medicine at the University of Pennsylvania School of Medicine and a world expert on the epidemiology of adverse drug reactions, encouraged the writing of this book and wrote the preface.

We also thank the many people at the Food and Drug Administration who provided information used in the book, and others who choose to remain anonymous.

Sidney M. Wolfe, M.D.
Chris Coley

November, 1980

CONTENTS

PREFACE

by
PAUL D. STOLLEY
Professor of Medicine
University of Pennsylvania
School of Medicine

An often-neglected aspect of a physician's training and continued education concerns the rational use of drugs. The task of updating physicians on drug prescribing after graduation has been largely assumed by the drug manufacturers themselves through conferences, journals, promotional materials and visits to physicians by drug company sales representatives. The information provided by drug manufacturers, while subject to Food and Drug Administration scrutiny and regulation, does not necessarily convey the attitudes of skepticism, objectivity, concern with consumer costs and choice of alternatives, including *no* drug therapy.

The Health Research Group has once again stepped into an area which has not received sufficient attention from the medical profession and academically-based pharmacologists to provide an up-to-date and balanced review of drugs used to treat many common disorders. Those drugs still available which lack conclusive (or even reasonably convincing) proof of their effectiveness are discussed and the efficacious and valuable drugs are highlighted to aid both patients and doctors.

This volume should prove useful to physicians in their everyday practice and medical students would profit from studying it and the critical way the drug literature is assessed. Most importantly, informed consumers will be able to protect themselves from risky and unproven drugs.

INDEX

Quinsone, *see F-E-P Creame,* pg. 101
Racet, *see Vioform-Hydrocortisone Mild,* pg. 187
Rate-10, *see Peritrate,* pg. 153
Rate 20, *see Peritrate,* pg. 153
Rate-T-30, *see Duotrate Plateau Caps,* pg. 96
Rautrax, pg. 165
Rautrax-N, pg. 167
Rautrax-N Modified, pg. 168
Rectacort Suppositories, *see Wyanoids HC Rectal Suppositories,* pg. 189
Reithritol, *see Peritrate,* pg. 153
Repan, pg. 168
Robinul-PH, pg. 169
Robinul-PH Forte, pg. 170
Roniacol, pg. 170
Roniacol Timespan Tabs, pg. 171
Ru-Vert, pg. 172
Scrip-Vasco, *see Nico-Metrazol,* pg. 133
Sedralex Elixir, *see Donnatal,* pg. 93
Sedralex Tablets, *see Donnatal,* pg. 93
Senilex, *see Nico-Metrazol,* pg. 133
Senilezol, *see Nico-Metrazol,* pg. 133
Senoral-M, *see Cenalene,* pg. 71
Setamine Liquid, *see Donnatal,* pg. 93
Setamine Tablets, *see Donnatal,* pg. 93
Sidonna, pg. 172
Sorate-2.5, *see Isordil Sublingual,* pg. 107
Sorate-5, *see Isordil Sublingual,* pg. 107
Sorate-10, *see Isordil Titradose,* pg. 108
Sorate-40, *see Isordil Tembids,* pg. 107
Sorbide T. D., *see Isordil Tembids,* pg. 107
Sorbide-10, *see Isordil Titradose,* pg. 108
Sorbitrate, *see Isordil Titradose and Chewable Tablets,* pg. 108
Sorbitrate SA, *see Isordil Tembids,* pg. 107
Sorbitrate Sublingual, *see Isordil Sublingual,* pg. 107
Spalix Elixir, *see Donnatal,* pg. 93
Spalix Tablets, *see Donnatal,* pg. 93
Spasmate, *see Pathibamate,* pg. 145
Spasmolin Capsules, *see Donnatal,* pg. 93
Spasmolin Tablets, *see Donnatal,* pg. 93
Spasmophen Elixir, *see Donnatal,* pg. 93
Spastyl, *see Bentyl,* pg. 59
Spastyl w/Phenobarbital, *see Bentyl w/Phenobarbital,* pg. 59
Spectrocin, pg. 173
Speniacol, *see Roniacol,* pg. 170
Spenpath, *see Pathibamate,* pg. 145

*This product is ineffective because of the time-release dosage form.

†After issuing its August 1, 1980 computer printout classifying drugs as effective and not effective, the FDA announced it was going to upgrade 15 drug products from "lacking substantial evidence of effectiveness" to "effective."[1] The 15 products are all ophthalmic (eye) drugs which are combinations of antibiotics and steroids. However, FDA officials have admitted that no studies have been submitted to prove the effectiveness of these products. They have also stated that the main reason for upgrading the drugs to "effective" was heavy pressure from eye doctors. The FDA's approval of these drugs is also inconsistent with the findings of the American Medical Association, which has concluded that these drugs are "irrational mixtures" and that they "are not recommended for the topical [local] treatment of ocular infections."[2]

The dangers of these drugs are discussed in the individual entries in this book. We continue to believe that these drugs are ineffective and dangerous and we strongly recommend against using them.

---

[1] Federal Register *45,* August 29, 1980, 57776.
[2] AMA Drug Evaluations (first edition, page 526), 1971.

Part I:
INTRODUCTION

You go to the doctor because you don't feel well. You are listened to (sometimes), examined, tested and then the doctor usually writes one or more prescriptions for you. You go to the drug store to have the prescription filled. You go home and start taking the pills. Now everything will be all right, right? Wrong.

Neither you nor, in some instances, even your doctor realizes that one out of every eight prescriptions filled—169 million prescriptions costing over $1.1 billion in 1979*—is for a drug not considered effective by the government's own standards. Since all drugs involve risks, this lack of effectiveness means you are exposing yourself to dangers without gaining compensating benefits. In other words, balancing the benefits versus the risks, these drugs are not safe. You have some questions?

Question: Why are these 607 drugs still on the market if they are not effective? Who says they are not effective?

Answer: In the mid to late 1960s the National Academy of Sciences-National Research Council on contract to the Food and Drug Administration (FDA) reviewed all prescription drugs marketed between 1938 and 1962 to determine if they complied with the 1962 drug amendments.

---

*1979 prescription and retail sales data *(National Prescription Audit: Therapeutic Category Report,* IMS America, Ambler, PA) for all drugs in this book for which figures were available.

1

This law required, for the first time, that drugs be proven effective with well-controlled studies. The FDA also conducted a major investigation which confirmed that thousands of drugs lacked evidence of effectiveness, but they delayed ordering many of the drugs removed from the market, particularly the big-selling drugs listed in this book (see 1979 Top 30 Less-Than-Effective Prescription Drugs, pg. 207). The FDA violated a court order that required the agency to have removed a large number of these drugs from the market by 1976 (see History section, pg. 193, for details). This book contains information on 607 drug products, each falling into one of the following categories:

1. —drugs that are listed in the FDA August 1980 computer printout of drugs lacking evidence of effectiveness and drugs identical in composition or related to these drugs but made by another company. These were reviewed by the National Academy of Sciences (NAS) and the FDA.

2. —additional drugs, although missing from the FDA computer printout, that have warning boxes on their labeling stating that the NAS has found that they lack evidence of effectiveness.

3. —drugs that contain *papaverine* or *ethaverine* and are sold to improve circulation in the head, limbs or heart. The FDA and an FDA advisory committee have both found that they lack evidence of effectiveness *and* of safety (see Papaverine and Ethaverine, pg. 27).

4. —drugs called vaginal sulfonamides which are used to treat vaginal infections. An FDA advisory committee concluded that these drugs also lack evidence of effectiveness (see AVC Cream, pg. 53).

5. —neomycin-containing drugs, used for direct application to the skin, which an FDA advisory committee on over-the-counter drugs has concluded lack evidence of effectiveness.

Question: Even though the FDA has failed to get these drugs off the market, why do doctors still prescribe ineffective drugs?

Answer: All these drugs have been on the market for at least 18 and often 25 or more years, and many physicians were in the habit of prescribing them before they were found to lack evidence of effectiveness. Even though the FDA requires labeling and advertising for many of these drugs to include a small box indicating the drugs lack evidence of effectiveness, many doctors pay as much attention to these little boxes as do smokers to the Surgeon General's warning box on cigarettes. Besides, many doctors think that if they judge a drug to work, even if scientific studies show it doesn't, they have the right to prescribe it. Early in the 1950's, DES (diethylstilbestrol) was shown in published, well-controlled studies not to protect women from miscarriage. Nevertheless, *after* this time, it was prescribed to prevent miscarriages in millions of women because some doctors "believed" the drug worked. Each had seen a woman with a miscarriage in a previous pregnancy take DES and avoid a miscarriage during a subsequent pregnancy. Blinded to the notion that it was not DES, but just the natural variation from one pregnancy to the next, doctors rejected scientific studies in deference to their own personal "experience" and therefore exposed millions of mothers, sons and daughters to DES, the effects of which have included cancer, birth defects and problems with pregnancies. In other words, DES as well as many of the drugs in this book are not only no more effective than but are also much more dangerous than a placebo (sugar pill).

Question: If a drug is not listed in this book, does it mean that the drug is O.K. to take?

Answer: No! This book lists only drugs or combinations of drugs that are not effective and that consequently provide risks without compensating benefits as of this writing. In addition, many drugs not listed here are very effective for certain serious diseases but are overprescribed for non-serious diseases such as colds. Antibiotics are a good example. When used inappropriately, these also subject patients to risks that outweigh the benefits. In addition, there are effective drugs that should not be given with other effective drugs because of dangerous interactions.

Question: What should I do if my doctor has prescribed one of the drugs listed in this book for me?

Answer: Ask your doctor if he or she knows the drug is considered to be ineffective (and/or dangerous) and why he or she prescribed it for you. Ask if there are alternatives (either another drug or a non-drug treatment) that would help your medical problem.

Question: Is it all right for patients to challenge doctors who prescribe drugs listed in this book?

Answer: Certainly. You will be doing yourself and the doctor a favor. By refusing to take such a drug, you will protect yourself from the needless risk of a bad reaction from a drug found not to be effective. You may also help the doctor because he or she too wants to avoid any bad reactions.

Question: Who else thinks people should not use these ineffective drugs even though they are still on the market?

Answer: 1. Former FDA Commissioner Dr. Donald Kennedy. In 1978 correspondence with other HEW officials about why ineffective drugs should not be paid for with federal Medicaid or Medicare funds, Dr. Kennedy said:

> the use of less-than-effective drugs may prolong therapy and result in increased patient discomfort as well as increased expense . . . the use of an irrational combination product (even though one ingredient may be effective) needlessly exposes the patient to the

risks of these ineffective components.
(See Combination Drug Products, below.)

2. Six states (Hawaii, Indiana, Iowa, Maryland, Nevada, New Mexico) and the District of Columbia do not now reimburse for many ineffective prescription drugs in their Medicaid programs.

3. U.S. Public Health Service hospitals and clinics do not use a large number of ineffective drugs.

4. Many good hospitals do not keep most ineffective drugs in their pharmacies.

Question: Will I always need this book?

Answer: No, but probably for at least four or five more years. The FDA will eventually ban most if not all of these drugs. In the interim, protect yourself and help your doctor.

WHAT ARE INEFFECTIVE DRUGS?

As of 1980, all of the 607 drug products listed in this book have been on the market for at least 18 years, most for 20, 30 years or more. Yet none of these drugs has been found by the U.S. Government to have substantial evidence of effectiveness in well-controlled studies. Another way these drugs are referred to is "less-than-effective," meaning that the government rated them only "probably effective," "possibly effective," or "ineffective" (see History section). All drugs in these three less-than-effective categories have never been proven effective by adequate well-controlled studies.

Since the legal standard is either effective or not effective and since the FDA has been removing drugs in all three less-than-effective categories from the market, we will use the phrase *ineffective* or *not effective* to refer to any drug that has not been found to have substantial evidence of effectiveness as of August 1980.

COMBINATION DRUG PRODUCTS

About two-thirds of the drug products in this book are fixed-ratio combinations. This means that these products combine two or more ingredients so that questions relating to their safety and efficacy depend not only on the safety and effectiveness of the individual drugs for specific symptoms, but also on the safety and efficacy of the drugs taken together. Some of the cough and cold preparations found in this guide, for example, contain as many as seven different drugs. Although the likelihood of unwanted side effects clearly increases proportionally with the number of drugs a person consumes, it is not true that increasing the number of different ingredients in a product will make that product better or more effective.

Some of these drugs do contain an effective ingredient and therefore may be of some therapeutic benefit if they are used. They are still considered ineffective, however, because one or more of their ingredients is ineffective. If the effective ingredient is needed, it should be taken alone because the combination is more potentially dangerous and at best no more effective than the single drug.

But there is another way of looking at what is wrong with combination drugs. If a drug preparation contains just one active ingredient, there is probably a 50% chance that the "average" dose will be appropriate for you. This is true because we all metabolize drugs at different rates. We also each metabolize different drugs at widely different rates. Suppose a drug preparation now contains two active ingredients, each alone possibly effective with a 50% chance in your case. The chance that *both* will be effective is 50% x 50% or 25%. If the drug contains three active ingredients, the chance that all three will be effective, using the same assumption, is only 12.5% or one out of eight.

In addition to former FDA Commissioner Kennedy's statement that "the use of an irrational combination product (even though one ingredient may be effective) needlessly exposes the patient to the risks of these ineffective components," many combination drugs have been explicitly cited as "irrational mixtures" by the *AMA Drug Evaluations* (first edition), a publication of the American Medical Association Council on Drugs. Also, when the United States Pharmacopeia selected only the best and proven drugs for which to set standards of strength, quality, and purity, combination drug products were excluded.

The Final Report of the National Academy of Sciences (NAS) Drug Efficacy Study in 1969 opposed combination drugs:

It is a basic principle of medical practice that more than one drug should be administered for the treatment of a given condition only if the physician is persuaded that there is substantial reason to believe that each drug will make a positive contribution to the effect he seeks. Risks of adverse drug reactions should not be multiplied *unless there be overriding benefit* (emphasis added). Moreover, each drug should be given at the dose level that may be expected to make its optimal contribution to the total effect, taking into account the status of the individual patient and any synergistic or antagonistic effects that one drug may be known to have on the safety or efficacy of the other. On these grounds, multiple therapy using fixed-dose ratios determined by the manufacturer and not by the physician is, in general, poor practice.

INEFFECTIVE DOSAGE FORMS— TIME-RELEASE

Some drugs listed in the book, including both combination drugs and single ingredient drugs, are effective in dosage forms such as tablets or capsules but, in a time-release dosage form, they lack evidence of effectiveness. Drugs of this type listed in the book will always have the ineffective dosage form listed in both the index and the drug listing.*

In general, the time-release dosage form is not effective because of uneven release of the active chemical over time, resulting in lower (or higher) levels of the drug getting absorbed into the blood stream from the intestinal tract.

IDENTICAL DRUGS

Many drugs in the index of this book do not have their own entries but instead refer the reader to another drug's entry. This is because the two drugs involved are "identical." They contain exactly the same active ingredients, have equal amounts of each ingredient and are administered in the same dosage form. In most cases only the drug with an actual entry has been officially found "less-than-effective" by the FDA. Since drugs listed as identical differ only in their inactive ingredients (i.e. the filler that holds together a tablet, capsule or syrup) they should be considered equally ineffective.

*Index entries for these drugs will have an asterisk next to the name of the drug product.

Part II:
TREATMENT FOR
COMMON DISEASES

INTRODUCTION TO TREATMENT FOR COMMON DISEASES

Of the 607 drugs in this book, most (three out of every four) belong to one of five different classes of drugs. These classes are:

Drugs for Cough, Cold and Allergy

Drugs for Heart Pain

Drugs for Circulatory Disorders of Head and Limbs

Drugs for Digestive Disorders

Drugs Applied Directly to Skin, Eye or Ear

In this part of the book, there is a case study for each of these five classes of drugs. The drugs in these five classes will either have an entry in Part III or will be referred to as a drug identical to an entry drug. Each entry will say "See Part II: Drugs for Cough, Cold and Allergy" or whichever class the drug belongs to. If the drug you want information about is, for example, ACTIFED, you would a) find the drug listed in the index, b) look up the entry on page 43 in Part III, and be told, at the end of the entry, to see Part II: Drugs for Cough, Cold and Allergy.

If, on the other hand, you looked up ACTAGEN in the index, it would say "see ACTIFED, pg. 43." This indicates that ACTAGEN and ACTIFED are drugs with identical active ingredients. You will then go through the process described above for ACTIFED.

Each case study begins with a summary of what the common disease is like, what treatments—drug or non-drug—are effective, and what is wrong with the pills that don't work in that class. The rest of the case study will describe the most common types of ingredients in the drugs in that class, how they are supposed to work, and some of their dangers as well as more details about information reviewed in the summary.

Five additional categories of ineffective drugs, each having fewer drugs than any of the above five case studies, are included in the book. For any drug in these five classes, in addition to the entry in Part III for the drug, you are referred to the entry for the most commonly prescribed drug in the class *(referral drug)* for more detailed information. These five classes, with the referral drug and its page number following in parentheses, are:

      —Vaginal Infections (AVC Cream, pg. 53)

      —Bone and Growth Disorders (Winstrol, pg. 188)

      —Central Nervous System Stimulants (Ru-Vert, pg. 172)

      —Combination Antibiotics (Mysteclin F, pg. 122)

      —Asthma Drugs (Marax, pg. 116)

For example, if you wanted information about a combination antibiotic such as ACHROSTATIN V, you would look it up in the index, read the entry on pg. 43 and, at the end of the entry, be referred to MYSTECLIN F, a similar drug, for a discussion on what is wrong with combination antibiotics.

Drugs for Cough, Cold and Allergy

Most coughs and colds are due to viruses, are uncomplicated and are self-limited. In other words, you usually get better in a week or less with or without drugs. Drinking lots of liquids, including soup and other hot beverages, and inhaling steam will help relieve cold symptoms.

Fever: Fever can be treated with *aspirin* or *acetaminophen.*

Cough: Coughing, especially if you are coughing something up, is a healthy way to clear your respiratory tract. Only if coughing is keeping you from sleeping should you consider using a cough medicine. Then, use *dextromethorphan,* available under the brand names Silence is Golden, Pertussin 8-Hour Cough Suppressant, Symptom I and Tricodene. If a cough lasts more than a week or if you are having difficulty breathing (shortness of breath) or chest pain with deep breathing or coughing, consult a nurse or doctor.

Runny Nose: Like coughing, a runny nose promotes drainage and should not be treated with medication.

Stuffy Nose: Only when your nose is blocked should you consider medication. A decongestant such as *phenylephrine* spray or drops can be used.

All of the above drugs are effective, are available over-the-counter, and are relatively inexpensive, especially if purchased in their generic form. There is no good evidence that antihistamines, effective for allergies such as hay fever, are helpful in treating colds. None of the 142 prescription cough, cold, and allergy products listed in this book—with retail sales of over 316 million dollars in 1979—are effective.

Prescription and over-the-counter (OTC) oral cough and cold drug products are big sellers in the United States market. There are more prescription products available for the treatment of cough and cold than for any other symptoms, and consumers purchased nearly $1 billion worth of these medications in 1979.[1]

Of the top 30 less-than-effective drugs, fourteen are in the cough, cold and allergy category. Unfortunately, many of these concoctions are on the market only because of FDA delays in banning them. Far from being the cure-all that drug companies would have you believe, most of these products are fixed-ratio combinations that fall far short of the manufacturer's claims.

All of the cough, cold and allergy products in this guide have been found by government panels of scientific experts to lack evidence of effectiveness; many of them contain four or more individual ingredients, some of which are ineffective and the use of which is irrational. Since no drug is entirely risk-free, the potential risk from a combination drug is significantly greater than from any of the ingredients taken alone. The various components may interact with one another to enhance toxicity, inhibit effectiveness, or simply expose the consumer to extra, unwanted side effects, often with no additional benefit.

Although this guide discusses ineffective prescription drugs, the following section also pertains to the thousands of OTC cough and cold products. "Many of these products are at best mostly useless, while many are harmful and some are even dangerous," said Senator Gaylord Nelson in his opening statement at the 1972 hearing on the safety and efficacy of cough and cold remedies.[2]

Cough Remedies

"Most coughs are associated with viral infections of the upper respiratory tract and these infections are usually self-limited, brief in duration and do not require medications. In fact, the cough reflex is a protective mechanism that helps rid the respiratory tract of secretions," according to *The New Handbook of Prescription Drugs.* The suppression of a "productive" cough, such as seen with pneumonia, thus prevents the removal of mucus and phlegm and may be dangerous.

In general, the two types of drugs used to treat coughs are *antitussives* and *expectorants.* Antitussives act in the brain to suppress the cough reflex. They include both narcotic agents (*codeine, hydrocodone*) and non-narcotic drugs *(dextromethorphan).* Some of the narcotic antitussives and similar drugs have significant pain-relieving and sedative action in addition to their cough-suppressing effects.

When coughing is especially bothersome, when little phlegm and mucus is present or when coughing becomes truly painful, dextromethorphan is the most appropriate drug. It is a non-narcotic and does not present the potential problems of abuse and physical dependence inherent in narcotic drugs such as codeine, although problems with codeine are rare if it is used correctly on a short-term basis. Dextromethorphan may be purchased as a *single-entity* product, that is to say, without all of the other drug agents that add nothing except cost, potential side effects and potential adverse reactions.

The other general class of drugs found in cough preparations, the expectorants, act peripherally, or "on-site." Manufacturers claim they help relieve coughing by thinning out the respiratory tract fluids so they can be more easily expelled. According to *AMA Drug Evaluations* (first edition, pg. 360), "[r]esults of clinical studies have generally shown no detectable decrease in sputum [phlegm] viscosity [thickness] or increase in sputum volume with the use of the expectorant agents. Thus, the efficacy of these agents used alone as antitussives and their usefulness in cough mixtures has not been fully defined." Besides demonstrating no convincing therapeutic benefit, virtually all of these expectorants have been associated with varying degrees of gastrointestinal disturbances. For example, *ammonium chloride,* found in a number of the ineffective cough mixtures in this guide (see, for example, *Ambenyl Expectorant*), is readily absorbed and, when given in large doses, produces a condition where the blood is abnormally acidic. Ammonium chloride could prove particularly hazardous in patients with improperly functioning lungs, liver or kidneys.

Another so-called expectorant found in a number of these multi-drug cough preparations is *ipecac fluid extract* (see the *Phenergan Expectorants*), a potent drug that has caused deaths in overdose and that should not be prescribed for treating coughs or any of the labeled indications associated with these drugs. The proper use of ipecac is to induce vomiting after poisoning and its presence in cough remedies is irrational and potentially hazardous.

One of the most commonly found expectorants in both prescription and OTC cough medicines is *guaifenesin (glyceryl guaiacolate).* It is claimed to act by stimulating secretion of respiratory tract fluid, thereby increasing the volume and decreasing the thickness of bronchial secretions. Few objective studies on its action are available, and its effectiveness is doubtful.

While the expectorants show little, if any, therapeutic value in cough medications, this doesn't mean they don't pose any risks to the patient. Many can cause serious, although infrequent, adverse reactions. Yet if they do not work as claimed, the relatively small risk from consuming them becomes significant. It becomes even more so when one considers that many of the cough medications sold today contain a number of these ineffective expectorants of dubious safety. *The Medical Letter,* a highly respected review of drug literature, has this to say about the multitude of cough concoctions available today: "…. there is no justification for using four or more drugs simultaneously, some having opposing effects on the cough reflex. Multiple fixed-ratio drugs also multiply adverse effects and prevent flexibility in dosages of the individual drugs."[3]

In sum, one should treat only the severe dry cough, and dextromethorphan is the most appropriate way to do this. This will avoid the problem of subjecting your body to a host of other medicines. If a severe cough persists for more than five to seven days, especially if it is accompanied by high fever, chest pain with deep breathing or coughing, or shortness of breath, consult a physician.

Cold Remedies

Acute infections of the upper respiratory tract are usually due to invading bacteria or viruses. However, symptoms are similar even when the cause varies. The burgeoning number of cold remedies, like those for cough (often products will claim to work for both), all focus on relieving the annoying symptoms, post-nasal drip, runny nose, nasal congestion, headache, body ache, malaise, cough and sometimes fever. At best, such an approach may make one more comfortable until the natural bodily defenders can bring about a full recuperation. However, as with any drug, risks are involved.

Some single-ingredient products provide effective symptomatic relief of the discomforts of the common cold: nasal decongestants, pain relievers (like aspirin), and antitussives (see Cough Remedies). However, no one agent can relieve all symptoms associated with the common cold; drug companies have become increasingly strident in marketing mixtures of drugs in fixed-ratio forms that are claimed to provide relief for every symptom. In virtually every case, these fixed-combinations are of little or no effectiveness. Many are irrational or even dangerous. According to the *AMA Drug Evaluations* (first edition, pg. 377), "[a]t best, they all have the principal disadvantage of fixed-dosage combination products, namely, that when a therapeutic amount of one agent is given, other drugs in the mixture may be administered at higher or lower levels than are optimally therapeutic. This disadvantage is particularly prominent with some of the cold remedies that are sold over-the-counter without prescription, for they may have been formulated to satisfy government safety requirements and contain certain ingredients in subtherapeutic quantities."

As with most of the cough preparations included in this guide, the products promoted and prescribed for the relief of cold symptoms are polydrug "shotgun" approaches. We believe that brand names containing such terms as "cold tablets" or "cold medicine" should be disallowed. Promotion should deal with specific symptoms, so that consumers will not expose themselves to unnecessary medication.

Decongestants

Decongestants are included in most of the popular prescription and OTC "cough and cold" medicines to prevent nasal dripping and unclog blocked sinus passages. One of the two most common types of decongestants is the vasoconstrictors (blood vessel constrictors), such as *phenylephrine* and *phenylpropanolamine*. Although the vasoconstricting agents might be effective if given in a sufficient dose (more than 40 milligrams or, preferably, given locally as in nosedrops) most of these prescriptions and OTC cold medications contain less than half that amount (*Dimetane* contains only 5 milligrams each of two common decongestants).

Oral vasoconstrictor drugs rarely do much to relieve nasal stuffiness. However, even if they were effective, they would still pose a real hazard for the 22 million Americans with high blood pressure, since vasoconstrictors can seriously aggravate this condition.[4] Furthermore, these agents are characterized quite often by a *rebound vasodilation.* In other words, when the effect of the drug wears off, the blood vessels of the sinus area expand more than ever to produce a new wave of congestion, and the individual then feels compelled to take another dose of the drug. A vicious cycle may develop through the overuse of this class of drugs. For a runny nose which is not stuffy, no drug treatment may be best since drainage can help clear up the infection.

Antihistamines

Antihistamines are good for allergies, not colds. Many of the ineffective cough and cold remedies in this guide contain one or more antihistamines, drugs that block the effects of the allergy chemical in the body, histamine, and thus alleviate the annoyances and discomfort of an allergic response. Antihistamines can have the effect of thickening bronchial secretions and thus act in opposition to expectorants that supposedly thin out secretions. Not only is there little evidence to substantiate their advertised usefulness for the "runny nose, sneezing, itching and watery eyes" of a cold, but there is also evidence to the contrary. Cough and cold medicine expert Dr. Phillip S. Norman,[5] Professor of Medicine, Johns Hopkins University, stated at Senator Nelson's hearings on cough and cold medicine:

> Careful comparisons between patients treated with antihistamines and patients treated with placebos [a sugar pill] showed no evidence that antihistamine usage either relieved the symptoms of a cold or shortened the duration of the illness.[6]

Dr. Richard Hornick, now Professor of Medicine, University of Rochester, stated at the same hearings:

> The rationale for the utilization of antihistamines is based on the fact that histamine is released in the process of certain types of inflammation. Thus, reactions due to antigen-antibody interactions [as in typical "allergic" reactions] release histamine.... However, in the type of inflammatory response occurring from a viral infection [as is the case with most colds] there is no evidence that there is a significant release of histamine.[7]

Their views were corroborated by other witnesses at the hearings: Dr. Jack M. Gwaltney, University of Virginia; Dr. Thomas W. Dunphy, Hunter Foundation for Health Care; Dr. Carl E. Arbesman, State University of Buffalo; and Dr. Sol Katz, Georgetown University—all experts in respiratory diseases.

Allowing the marketing of antihistamines for unproven benefits, such as the treatment of colds, is unsafe because of their side effects: drowsiness (sometimes quite prominent, which is why certain antihistamines are often employed as sleeping aids), uncoordination, mental inattention and dizziness. This can be a problem for a person not resting in bed. Blood disorders have also been reported with antihistamine use on rare occasions.

The possible toxicity of the antihistamine promethazine (jaundice, decreased production of white blood cells, rashes) argues against its use in minor illnesses. As the *AMA Drug Evaluations* (third edition, pg. 1104) states, promethazine "can produce any of the adverse reactions observed with other phenothiazines." Although none of the phenothiazine drugs (most are sold as tranquilizers) appear to be completely free of the risk of complications affecting the nervous system (extrapyramidal stimulation) which is being recognized more frequently, especially in older patients, "promethazine is relatively free of . . . extrapyramidal stimulation" (Ibid). While adverse reactions are less likely to happen with only occasional use of promethazine-containing drugs like *Phenergan Expectorant,* taking these drugs presents a potentially serious and clearly unnecessary risk. Doctors should realize that promethazine in these products confers no counter-balancing medical benefit to the patient.

This is not to say that antihistamines have no place at all in drug prescribing. When used in single-entity preparations at the correct dosage, these agents are very useful for genuine allergic conditions, such as hay fever or hives.

Secretion Inhibitors (Anticholinergics)

Some of the cold remedies in this guide attempt to dry up nasal and throat secretions by including agents that act not only to block histamine but inhibit a certain set of cell components called *cholinergic receptors.* These receptors are responsible for all sorts of bodily secretions. Some of the specific *anticholinergic* agents are the *belladonna alkaloids, atropine* (a particular component of belladonna), *isopropamide iodide* (found in *Ornade)* and *homatropine* (found in *Hycodan*). These anticholinergic agents have significant action at the level of the gastrointestinal tract, exerting antispasmodic and antisecretory effects; you will also find these agents in many of the less-than-effective products employed for various digestive disorders. Adverse reactions may be severe at excessive dosage levels. Moreover, by including these anticholinergic "drying" agents in multidrug formulations containing expectorants that supposedly act to increase secretions, many drug companies have succeeded in creating "irrational" products. Not only do many of the individual ingredients counteract each other (as in Ambenyl Expectorant), they also greatly increase the risk of adverse reactions without providing additional therapeutic benefit. If a drug is desired, treat the worst of the "cold" symptoms, such as "runny nose," with single-entity drug products (all available OTC). Avoid the expensive, potentially harmful and essentially ineffective "shotgun" cough and cold combinations.

Recommended therapy for individual cold or cough symptoms is:

—*Stuffy Nose:* Phenylephrine hydrochloride in nose drop or spray form, either generically or in brand name form such as Neo-Synephrine.

—*Runny Nose:* Like coughing, a runny nose promotes drainage and should not be treated with medication.

—Headache, Body Ache: Aspirin or acetaminophen. Tylenol is one of several brands of acetaminophen.

—Fever: Aspirin or acetaminophen.

—Cough: If dry, hacking cough is present, treat with dextromethorphan, available as Silence is Golden, Pertussin 8-Hour Cough Suppressant, Symptom I or Tricodene. Productive cough should not be treated.

Finally, a few of the cough preparations found in this guide contain alcohol (such as Benylin Cough Syrup and Phenergan Expectorant). The practice of lacing these remedies with alcohol is even more prevalent among the OTC products (such as Nyquil, 25 percent or 50 proof). In the case of fixed-combination drug mixtures containing alcohol, there is positive evidence of a heightened effect with ingredients such as antihistamines to cause drowsiness. This can be dangerous, especially if one has to remain alert, such as when driving a car. Alcohol also adds to the effects of tranquilizers and some pain relievers, like codeine. There is no evidence that alcohol has any therapeutic benefit in relieving the symptoms of cough and cold, yet many such products especially those sold OTC contain it.

FOOTNOTES

[1] *National Prescription Audit,* IMS America, Ambler, PA, 1979.

[2] Hearings of the Senate Subcommittee on Monopoly of the U.S. Senate Small Business Committee. Advertising of Proprietary Medicines. 3:939, 1972.

[3] *The Medical Letter.* 13:9-11, 1971.

[4] Graedon J. *The People's Pharmacy.* St. Martin's Press. p. 65, 1976.

[5] Dr. Norman served on the NAS-NRC Drug Review that became the basis for the FDA DESI project.

[6] Testimony presented to Senate Subcommittee on Monopoly of the U.S. Senate Small Business Committee. Advertising of Proprietary Medicines. 3:1012, 1972.

[7] *Ibid.,* 982.

Drugs for Heart Pain

The initial treatment of *angina pectoris* (transient heart pain due to inadequate blood supply to the heart) involves proper weight control, rest, cessation of smoking, treatment of hypertension if it exists, the use of nitroglycerin under the tongue for relief of acute pain or prevention of pain from exertion shortly after use, and the avoidance of sudden strenuous physical activity to which the person has not become conditioned. However, gradually increasing daily exercise under supervision may be helpful in increasing exercise tolerance.

For some patients, a newer drug, *propranolol* (brand name *Inderal*), has provided an additional degree of relief if the above measures do not work. Propranolol has been found very useful in diminishing the frequency and severity of anginal pain in many patients suffering from this condition. However, it cannot prevent such pain from occurring altogether. And, once an attack begins, this drug is not effective for relieving it. There also are potential serious side effects associated with this drug, including worsening of asthma and heart failure. So, while propranolol can be a useful drug for treating angina, it is by no means risk-free.

A 2% ointment of *nitroglycerin* (such as *Nitro-Bid*) applied to the skin has been found effective, in a recent properly-controlled study, in protecting against anginal attacks. High doses (at least 120 mg per day) of *isosorbide dinitrate* (as in *Isordil Tembids*) have also been recently found effective in preventing anginal attacks. Both these drugs are currently thought by the FDA to lack substantial evidence of effectiveness—but this is under review.

Coronary artery disease is a major health problem in the United States today, but despite extensive medical and scientific research, the underlying causes remain poorly understood. Post-mortem examinations have shown that by twenty-two years of age, 50 percent of American military casualties have gross evidence of *atherosclerosis* (variable degrees of clogged arteries). By age fifty, the incidence rises to over 90 percent, and nearly 50 percent have marked narrowing of one or more of the *coronary* arteries (blood vessels which supply blood to the heart itself).[1]

Atherosclerosis decreases blood flow, and when flow becomes inadequate to meet the demand for blood, symptoms result. Among the outstanding symptoms is heart pain (angina pectoris) in the case of coronary artery involvement and leg pain in the case of peripheral blood vessel disease (see Drugs for Circulatory Disorders of Head and Limbs). Angina pectoris* is a transient squeezing, heavy pain or ache in the chest, sometimes also felt in the neck and other areas of the upper body. Angina is often brought on by physically strenuous activity, such as shovelling snow.

Since the prognosis for long-term survival is not good once disease of the coronary vessels becomes symptomatic (painful), one of the principal goals must be the primary prevention of coronary disease.[2]

A number of risk factors in the development of coronary artery disease have been discovered. The main ones are high blood pressure (hypertension), smoking, high blood cholesterol level, diabetes, obesity, family history of coronary artery disease and sedentary living.

Identification of these factors has led to the hypothesis, but not to the firm conclusion, that the control of these risk elements may decrease the incidence of heart disease. Evidence strongly indicates that people who quit smoking improve their chances when compared to smokers. There is also mounting evidence that control of moderate to severe high blood pressure lowers the risk of heart attack (myocardial infarction) and definitely lowers the risk of stroke. There is a strong correlation between markedly elevated serum cholesterol and the risk of coronary artery disease. Cholesterol levels *can* be lowered by diet—and in such patients it appears to warrant the effort. In addition, gradually increasing daily exercise under medical supervision can improve the exercise tolerance level of patients with coronary artery disease allowing them to increase the amount of physical exercise they can perform before experiencing anginal pain.

---

*Angina pectoris (transient pain episodes) must be clearly distinguished from the pain associated with a myocardial infarction (heart attack) which ordinarily persists much longer.

How Heart Pain Drugs Are Supposed to Work and Why Their Effects Are Hard to Evaluate

Exactly how angina occurs when there is not enough oxygen to supply the heart muscle is unknown. Most *antianginal* drugs are also called *coronary vasodilators* on the assumption that they relieve this pain by dilating the coronary arteries. This assumption is only partially correct. Current evidence indicates that a reduction in the oxygen requirement of the heart muscle may account for the therapeutic action of the drugs.[3] Usually anginal pain disappears quickly with rest, which reduces oxygen requirements; therefore it is often not clear whether the drug or the rest relieved the pain.

In assessing the value of antianginal agents, it is important to differentiate between drugs used for the treatment or preventive management of an *acute* attack (sharp, with rapid onset) and those used for *long-term* prevention of these attacks. The efficacy of therapy for actually preventing or diminishing the frequency and severity of anginal attacks is difficult to evaluate because the frequency, duration, and severity of attacks vary and may be influenced by external factors (e.g. weather, anxiety, physical exertion) and because any antianginal effect is quite subjective.

Vasodilator Drugs: Nitrates

Nitroglycerin is the prototype *organic nitrate* vasodilator used to treat patients with an attack of angina pectoris. The mechanism of action of this drug remains unclear. However, when taken sublingually (under the tongue), nitroglycerin is the preferred drug for the *short-term* treatment and preventive management of acute attacks.

Nitroglycerin ointment can also provide up to several hours of protection against anginal attacks as shown in a recent well-controlled study.[4] At present, however, the FDA rates nitroglycerin ointment as lacking substantial evidence of effectiveness.

Lower doses of isosorbide dinitrate—as in Isordil—lack evidence of therapeutic effectiveness in preventing angina. In one recent report, however, extremely high doses of isosorbide dinitrate, administered for one month, were shown in a well-conducted study to be able to increase exercise tolerance for as long as six hours after administration and to decrease the frequency of anginal attacks during the one month period.[5] The authors are careful to state, however, that "administration of capsules of isosorbide dinitrate, *in the dosage utilized in the present study,* was of value in the prophylactic treatment of angina pectoris" (emphasis added). The dosage used was one 40 milligram capsule every 8 hours or 120 milligrams a day. But at present only a tiny fraction of all patients taking drugs containing isosorbide dinitrate are getting a dose as large as the one found effective in the study just mentioned.

In 1979, for example, there were 9.4 million prescriptions filled for various forms of isosorbide dinitrate. But only 1.1 million or 12% of the prescriptions were for the 40 milligram size and even those had an average daily dose of only 2 pills per day (80 mg) or two-thirds of that found effective (120 mg) in the one study discussed above.[6] Thus, it is likely that over 95% of patients getting isosorbide are getting a daily dose of less than the amount shown effective in this one study. As with nitroglycerin ointment, isosorbide is presently found lacking substantial evidence of effectiveness by the FDA. But the more recent study is currently under review.

Most of the other coronary vasodilator products included in this book—all given less-than-effective evaluations by the National Academy of Sciences-National Research Council (NAS-NRC)—are of the *orally* administered "long-acting" nitrate variety, such as *pentaerythritol tetranitrate (Peritrate), erythritol tetranitrate (Cardilate), mannitol hexanitrate* and nitroglycerin (oral, time-release form). These drugs have been ineffective in the preventive management of angina pectoris. The main problem with these so-called "long-acting" nitrates is that up to now most have neither been shown to be effective nor very long-acting. Most published studies demonstrate that their vasodilating effect lasts for 45 minutes to one hour, only slightly longer than the effects of sublingual nitroglycerin.[7] The results of some studies have revealed that at the doses usually given, these orally administered agents are rapidly destroyed by the liver before they can even reach the coronary vessels.[8]

Other Drugs for Heart Pain Which Are Not Effective

In addition to the antianginal oral nitrates, this guidebook includes certain non-nitrate drug products which are also used in the treatment of angina pectoris. They are *dipyridamole (Persantine),* a so-called "long-lasting" coronary vasodilator, and a large number of *papaverine* (see *Pavabid*) and *ethaverine* (see *Ethatab*) products (see Drugs for Circulatory Disorders of Head and Limbs).

Although Persantine does increase the coronary blood flow in animal studies, controlled double-blind studies (where neither the investigator nor the subject knows which kind of treatment is being given, in order to eliminate observer and subject bias) in man have demonstrated that this agent does not significantly decrease the incidence or severity of anginal attacks. Persantine has not been proven effective in the prevention or long-term treatment of angina.

Since papaverine and ethaverine do directly relax and dilate the coronary arteries in *normal* animals, the use of these drugs has been advocated to decrease the incidence of anginal attacks. However, convincing evidence of their effectiveness is lacking; what is more, liver toxicity has been associated with their use.[9] Actually, most of the prescriptions for these drugs are written for circulatory disorders of the limbs or brain for which these drugs are also not effective. Their use among anginal patients is less prevalent and appears to be diminishing.

FOOTNOTES

[1] *Federal Register.* 37:26624, December 14, 1972.
[2] Melmon KL, Morrelli HF. *Clinical Pharmacology,* 2nd ed., 284, 1978.
[3] *AMA Drug Evaluations,* 2nd ed., 21, 1973.
[4] Davidov ME, Mroczek WJ. *Angiology.* 27:205-211, 1976.
[5] Lee G, Mason DT, Amsterdam EA, Miller RR, DeMaria AN. *Chest.* 73:327-32, 1978.
[6] *National Prescription Audit,* IMS America, Ambler, PA, 1979.
[7] Melmon KL, Morrelli HF. *Clinical Pharmacology,* 2nd ed., 291, 1978.
[8] Coffman JD. *N Eng J Med* 300:713-717, 1979.
[9] Ronnov-Jessen V, Tjerlund A. *N Eng J Med* 281:1333-35, 1969.

Drugs for Circulatory Disorders of Head and Limbs

Drugs that allegedly increase poor blood circulation by direct or indirect dilating action on the peripheral (arms and legs) and cerebral (brain) blood vessels are called *vasodilators*. These products are widely advertised in medical journals and sales account for tens of millions of dollars of drug company profits each year. While it is true that most vasodilating drugs do increase the blood flow to the head and limbs in the *normal* human being, there is no acceptable evidence that such drugs produce a clinically important benefit, such as the relief of leg pain in patients with peripheral blood vessel disease or the reduction in dementia in patients with cerebral vascular disease.[1] These problems are often due to atherosclerosis or hardening of the arteries.

Eighty percent of prescriptions for these so-called circulation-improving drugs are written for people 65 and older.[2] Thus, drug companies are exploiting millions of older people with drugs that do not work, are expensive (retail sales of $111 million in 1979 for 10.5 million prescriptions filled) and cause a variety of adverse reactions. One such harmful effect—liver damage—is estimated to occur in about 20% of people taking papaverine drugs (see last part of this section).

Two articles, one on limb blood vessel disease and one on blood vessel disease of the head, summarize the present state of affairs.[3,4] After describing why vasodilator drugs are not effective for treating poor circulation of the limbs, the author says that "the most important aspects in the management include control of weight and blood lipids [fat]; prophylactic foot care; exercise, and consideration of bypass surgery for non-healing skin lesions [ulcers], rest pain [pain without walking], or disabling claudication." A recent editorial in the *British Medical Journal,* discussing cerebral vasodilator drugs for senile dementia, said these drugs have "no place" and that, "[i]ndeed by making the doctor feel that he is doing something, the administration of these drugs may actually deflect him from really important tasks: providing the patient and family with sympathy, practical advice and support."[5]

Blood Vessel Disease—Limbs

For therapeutic purposes, peripheral vascular diseases can be generally classified into two types: *obstructive* and *vasospastic.* Examples of the obstructive type include *arteriosclerosis obliterans* (a disease of the arteries characterized by thickening of the inner wall and obstruction of blood flow) and *intermittent claudication* (cramp-like leg pain and weakness often precipitated by exercise and associated with blood vessel spasm and obstruction). The most common example of vasospastic disease (involving blood vessel constriction) is Raynaud's disease (cold, discolored feet and hands due to constricted blood vessels).

In a recent article published in the *New England Journal of Medicine,* Dr. Jay D. Coffman found that, except for the use of *tolazoline (Priscoline)* in the treatment of vasospastic disease (Raynaud's), the peripheral vasodilator drugs included in this guide have no substantial evidence to justify their use in peripheral vascular disease.[1]

Coffman points out that while tolazoline (Priscoline) is of no benefit in treating obstructive arterial disease, it is "occasionally useful" in patients with Raynaud's disease when taken in combination with other agents. However, it is not the drug of choice for this condition (*guanethidine* is preferred) and, at present, the government thinks it is lacking substantial evidence of effectiveness even for this condition. Furthermore, the number of prescriptions of Priscoline written for Raynaud's disease represents only one percent of the total number written each year.[2] The vast majority of the prescriptions for tolazoline (Priscoline) are for obstructive peripheral arterial disease and for so-called cerebrovascular disease.

In obstructive arterial disease, the blood circulation beyond the point of narrowing or occlusion depends almost exclusively on smaller vessels in the immediate vicinity, so-called *collaterals,* which detour blood around the blocked or constricted area. Beyond the point of obstruction the circulation and blood pressure are diminished. It has been found that during exercise the pressure from the contracting muscle in the affected area on the blood vessel can exceed the pressure inside the vessel, markedly decreasing or even cutting off local circulation altogether. The dilation of blood vessels beyond the point of obstruction will not improve blood flow or raise the local blood pressure unless the obstruction is by-passed by dilating the surrounding vessels (collaterals). One of the best ways to accomplish this is to *increase* the general body blood pressure. Unfortunately, most vasodilator drugs tend to *decrease* body blood pressure, and none has been shown to dilate the collateral vessels.[1]

If one were trying to design the perfect drug for the treatment of peripheral vascular diseases, one would want the drug to dilate vessels and improve blood flow only in those areas where blood supply is deficient. At this point, such a drug doesn't exist. As has been pointed out by medical experts on this subject, in some circumstances the existing peripheral vasodilators, by causing vasodilation in other areas of the body without diseased vessels, may actually "steal" blood flow from the affected area. There is less resistance to blood flow in vasodilated areas than in a limb supplied by smaller, collateral blood vessels. Since flow follows the path of least resistance, blood goes to the normal areas and gets shunted away from the diseased limb. Adverse effects can be frequent and unpleasant. They include headache, nausea, chills, flushing, tingling and burning sensation of the skin (especially the scalp), heart flutter and gastrointestinal disturbances. Thus, instead of providing therapeutic benefit, there is growing evidence that these peripheral vasodilator drugs may injure the patient.[3]

Obstructive peripheral vascular disease (atherosclerosis) is a major health problem today. However, the FDA's Director of the Bureau of Drugs admits that at present "there are no drugs rated as effective for symptoms due to peripheral vascular disease."[6] Yet the FDA's rationale has been that because Americans *need* oral drugs to deal with peripheral vascular disease, they will allow these ineffective drugs to be marketed since there is no better alternative. The fact remains that these drugs simply do not work, and no amount of time extensions, procrastination and further clinical studies are going to change that fact.

Blood Vessel Disease—Head

Vasodilator drugs are also not considered useful in treating disease thought to be due to obstructed or constricted blood vessels in the brain. Many doctors prescribe these general peripheral vasodilators (including *papaverine* and *ethaverine*) for "senility", a term which says little, if anything, about the underlying physical disorder. Of the more than three million persons over the age of 65 afflicted with symptoms of brain disorders, it has been estimated that 20% suffer from treatable conditions, such as *hypothyroidism.*[7] Physicians have often dismissed the symptoms of brain dysfunction in old age as inevitable and irreversible. However, there is growing awareness that senility is not the inevitable outcome of aging, and in fact, is not even a disease but rather a term frequently used to describe a large number of conditions with an equally large number of causes. *Dementia* in the elderly has been called *senile dementia, senility* and *hardening of the arteries,* among other names. Dementia and organic brain syndrome are equivalent terms, indicating a decline in mental functioning as measured by impairment of memory, orientation, calculation, learning ability, and analytic power.

Admittedly, the majority of people with symptoms of dementia suffer from an irreversible condition of one sort or another. Yet, it is estimated that some three hundred thousand persons can be restored to useful life by appropriate evaluation and treatment. However, the use of vasodilators is not among treatments with proven therapeutic value. The irreversible cases of senility are sometimes called *primary* dementia to emphasize that the underlying problem lies with the brain cells themselves, whereas the reversible treatable cases are called *secondary* dementia to stress that the primary or underlying disease process is not in the brain cells themselves but is exerting a secondary, harmful effect on the brain. A good example of secondary dementia is that induced by a drug or by emotional depression. Depression as a cause of intellectual impairment, and hence senility, in older people is often overlooked by doctors despite mounting evidence that depression is a common response to crises occurring in later life.

Most people with so-called primary dementia, i.e., an irreversible condition acting at the level of the brain cells themselves, suffer from one of two particular disorders: *Alzheimer's disease* or *multiple infarct dementia.* Alzheimer's disease is characterized by a progressive degeneration of the brain tissue, especially those areas involved with memory and intellectual thought. As far as we know, the cause of this condition has nothing to do with inadequate blood supply and there is neither a rational basis nor clinical evidence for the use of vasodilator drugs in patients with

Alzheimer's disease.

The other major irreversible primary dementia, called multiple infarct dementia, involves multiple areas of cerebral softening and dead brain tissue and is associated with significant reduction in blood circulation to these areas. There is strong evidence that this problem is primarily the result of obstruction in the small arteries of the brain, *arteriosclerosis* (hardening of the arteries) and hypertension. There is no satisfactory clinical evidence that vasodilating drugs are of any therapeutic value to patients in prevention or cure of this condition.

Papaverine and Ethaverine

In 1962, when Congress passed amendments containing the new drug provisions to the federal Food, Drug and Cosmetic Act, they required that all drugs licensed between 1938 and 1962 be reviewed for effectiveness (see History section for more details). Under a "grandfather clause" included in the Act, drugs marketed prior to 1938 continued to be regulated under the Food and Drug Act of 1906. To gain exemption under this clause, manufacturers had to show that an identical drug, in the same dosage form and with the exact same labeled uses was introduced on the market prior to 1938. However, the Food and Drug Administration has ruled that none of the manufacturers of the 55 currently marketed brand-name products containing *papaverine* or *ethaverine* have qualified for the grandfather exemption. Since they also have not qualified for a license, the sale of their drugs appears to be blatantly illegal. None of these products were included in the National Academy of Sciences-National Research Council (NAS-NRC) evaluation and hence none of these drugs are formally part of the drug efficacy review project.

Papaverines and ethaverines basically have identical actions: ethaverine is just a synthetic derivative of papaverine which is twice as potent. These drugs are claimed to improve circulation by dilating blood vessels. They are promoted for blood vessel diseases associated with insufficient blood flow resulting from either blocked arteries or blood vessel spasms. They are most often used to treat symptoms in the head or limbs and less often to treat heart pain due to poor circulation. The manufacturers claim these drugs have special efficacy in preserving blood circulation to the brain, preventing vessel constriction that might result in brain damage and relieving and reducing symptoms after damage occurs. Their sales are booming because doctors feel pressured to provide "tangible" therapy for elderly patients with mental difficulties. But in 1973, the American Medical Association evaluated these drugs and concluded that there was no convincing evidence that papaverines have any therapeutic value for the above problems.[8] In 1976, fourteen years after the passage of the 1962 drug amendments, the FDA first stated that the evidence for the claims made with respect to these products was questionable. In order to determine the validity of these claims, the FDA at that time requested data on safety and effectiveness from manufacturers. In 1979, the FDA finished studying the data and published its findings, stating that "there are no adequate and well-controlled clinical investigations conducted by experts ... which provide substantial evidence of the effectiveness of these drugs. In addition, the agency is not aware of any evidence establishing the safety of the drugs for their indicated uses."[9] This notice went on to say that none of these drugs should be exempted from review under the grandfather clause.[10] An FDA Advisory Committee held hearings in mid-1979 to gather additional evidence about these drugs. The Committee unanimously concluded that "there is no body of evidence that will support the effectiveness of papaverine and ethaverine for any of the claimed indications."[11]

These drugs are not only ineffective; they are clearly dangerous. In 1969, 20% of patients receiving a moderate dose of papaverine (160 milligrams a day) for more than one month were found to have liver damage caused by the drug.[12] The authors of this study, remarking at how surprising it was that this had not been seen earlier, concluded that it was probably because papaverine "has long been considered a non-toxic drug." In an accompanying editorial, world expert on drug-induced liver damage Dr. Hyman Zimmerman said "If the therapeutic role of papaverine were important, the apparent hepatoxicity[liver toxicity]might be acceptable. Otherwise, perhaps its use should be abandoned, especially if other clinics find evidence of hepatic [liver] injury."[13] Such evidence has been found.

There are currently 55 brand name products on the market with papaverine or ethaverine as their active ingredient. These products accounted for 5.2 million prescriptions and $47 million in sales in 1979. The most popular brand is *Pavabid*, with sales over $31 million in 1979.[14] Ethaverine is most commonly purchased as *Ethatab* or *Ethaquin*.

There is no excuse for the fourteen year delay between the passing of the 1962 drug amendments and the FDA's first action in 1976. Equally inexcusable is the four year further delay in removing these ineffective and dangerous drugs from the market. Based on the available evidence, there is no reason to be using any ethaverine-papaverine-based product.

FOOTNOTES

[1] Coffman JD. *New Eng J Med.* 300: 713-717, 1979.

[2] *National Disease and Therapeutic Index,* I.M.S. America, Ambler, PA, 1975.

[3] Intermittent Claudication. *American Family Physician,* June, 1979.

[4] Naide D. *American Family Physician,* 22: 128-129, 1980.

[5] *British Medical Journal,* Editorial. 2:511-512, 1979.

[6] *Federal Register.* 37:26624, December 14, 1972. Restated in a 1977 letter from Dr. J. Richard Crout, Director of the Food and Drug Administration Bureau of Drugs, to Michael Harper, Esq., Center for Law and Social Policy, Washington, DC.

[7] Besdine R. *Treatable Dementia in the Elderly.* Task Force Draft presented at NIH Consensus Development Conference on Treatable Brain Diseases in the Elderly, July, 1978.

[8] *AMA Drug Evaluations,* 2nd ed., 30, 1973.

[9] *Federal Register.* 44:22193, April 13, 1979.

[10] *Federal Register.* 44:22181, April 13, 1979.

[11] *FDA Drug Bulletin,* November, 1979.

[12] Ronnov-Jessen V, Tjernlund A. *New Eng J Med.* 281: 1333-35 and 1364-65 1969.

[13] Zimmerman HJ. *New Eng J Med.* 281:1364-65, 1969.

[14] *National Prescription Audit,* I.M.S. America, Ambler, PA, 1979.

Drugs for Digestive Disorders

The 55 drug products in this book called sedative-gastrointestinal combinations all contain two kinds of drugs. The sedative ingredient is either a barbiturate such as *phenobarbital* or a tranquilizer whose implicit purpose is to calm the person and therefore calm the gastrointestinal tract. The gastrointestinal ingredient—whose purpose is to directly calm the stomach and intestines—is an *antispasmodic* drug, also called *anticholinergic* or *antisecretory*. Although such combination drugs are supposed to treat the symptoms caused by ulcers or other stomach or intestinal problems such as irritable bowel, for none of them is there evidence that the combination is more effective than the proper dose of the stomach/intestinal-calming ingredient alone or an antacid alone. According to *AMA Drug Evaluations* (third edition, pg. 1054), "most combination products do not provide an adequate amount of either anticholinergic agent or sedative."

In addition to the 55 sedative-gastrointestinal combination products, there are 11 gastrointestinal products without sedatives which also lack evidence of effectiveness. In 1979, Americans filled 25 million prescriptions for these ineffective drugs at a retail cost of 152 million dollars.

Antispasmodics

The primary use of antispasmodics is to relieve spasms in muscles of the gastrointestinal tract. They block the action of the natural chemical acetylcholine, which causes smooth muscle contractions, and are therefore also called anticholinergics. They also have antisecretory effects; they decrease the rate of acid secretion in the stomach. However, at the same time, they cause symptoms such as dry mouth, rapid heart beat, constipation and difficulty and hesitancy of urination. Examples of antispasmodics include *belladonna, atropine, scopolamine, propantheline, clidinium* and *isopropamide.*

Sedatives/Tranquilizers

These ingredients are added to the antispasmodic ingredient with the thought that calming the brain will indirectly calm the stomach and intestines. As mentioned above, no evidence exists showing that the addition of sedatives or tranquilizers to antispasmodics improves the efficacy of an adequate dose of the antispasmodic alone.

Examples of the sedative or tranquilizer component of these combination drugs include *chlordiazepoxide, meprobamate, hydroxyzine, prochlorperazine* and barbiturates such as *phenobarbital* and *butabarbital.* The barbiturates, in addition to their sedative properties, may cause addiction if used over an extended period of time.

A strongly-worded condemnation of these combination products is found in the *AMA Drug Evaluations* (first edition, pg. 593) which said:

There are many widely-promoted mixtures containing antispasmodics in fixed combination with other drugs such as barbiturates, antianxiety agents, phenothiazines, or antacids.*Such mixtures are irrational and are not recommended* because the dose of each agent should be individually adjusted to the patient and because of the possibility that such combinations might produce undesired drug interactions ... [and] patients requiring large doses of the antispasmodic would be bothered by the sedative effect of the other ingredients. [Emphasis added.]

Drugs Applied Directly to Skin, Eye or Ear

Diseases of the skin, eye or ear may be due to infections. If there is a serious infection, the proper effective antibiotic (usually given orally or by injection) should be used. Steroids—drugs which are useful for treating non-infected skin (such as in severe poison ivy)—should not be used. Using steroids for infections can be dangerous because they can either mask the evidence of infection or impair the body's defense system and increase the chance of worsening the skin infection. Sixty of the 72 drugs for skin, eye and ear in this book contain both an antibiotic (antibacterial or antifungal) and a steroid, implying they are intended for treatment of infection but adding the dangers of a steroid.

Without antibiotics, the chance of infection in minor cuts and wounds is relatively small. When infections do occur, they can usually be handled by the body's normal healing apparatus aided by washing the affected area with soap. For those skin, eye or ear problems in which there is no evidence of an infection, using an antibiotic does not make any sense. However, many of these 72 products are prescribed by doctors who, unable to make a proper diagnosis, prescribe a multiple ingredient drug to cover all bets.

In 1979, consumers filled 18 million prescriptions for these skin, eye or ear products at a retail cost of 116 million dollars.

Some 72 products in this guide are promoted and sold for external applications to the skin, eye or ear. Among the ointments, creams and solutions available, 31 contain *neomycin sulfate,* an antibiotic, which is potentially dangerous when used in this manner. In eleven of these drugs neomycin is mixed with one or two of the other antibiotics. In addition, 25 products combine neomycin with steroid drugs. Some of these are available only by prescription and others are available over the counter (OTC) as well.

Like all antibiotics, neomycin is used to treat infection. But there is little evidence to warrant the manufacturers' contention that applying antibiotics such as neomycin to skin infections is effective therapy. In many instances, it may actually be harmful. It commonly causes skin rashes; tests have demonstrated that such drug reactions appear in 49 percent of persons with previous skin problems, and in up to eight percent of those with no history of skin trouble.[1] Neomycin can cause uncomfortable allergic reactions such as inflammation, scaling, itching and blistering of the skin. It can sensitize the skin to effects from chemicals structurally related to neomycin such as some other antibiotics which, unlike neomycin, actually work.[2, 3]

For the treatment of serious skin or ear infections, most medical experts recommend giving the appropriate antibiotic either orally or by injection after a culture has identified the cause. But consumers should not expose themselves to any antibiotic for so-called "prevention" of minor skin infections. Without these products, the chance of infection in minor cuts and wounds is relatively small. But when infections do in fact occur, they can usually be handled by the body's normal healing apparatus aided by washing the affected area with soap. For none of the individual antibiotic agents in these topical products is there evidence that the preventive agent is the antibiotic rather than the physical barrier provided by the ointment base alone, or that the agent prevents infection at all.

When disease-causing bacteria are repeatedly attacked by a certain antibiotic, strains can develop that are resistant to the antibiotic. Unnecessary exposure to antibiotics is harmful because it increases the chance of resistant bacteria developing. Antibiotics to which bacteria are resistant are useless for the treatment of serious infection. Strains of infection-causing bacteria have developed that are resistant to neomycin.[4] Bacteria that become resistant to neomycin may be resistant to the related antibiotic *kanamycin,* which is used to treat serious infections, and are likely resistant to other important, structurally related drugs such as *gentamicin.*[5] The FDA report states: "Topical application of neomycin throughout the population could potentially play a role in the increase of resistant organisms, not just to neomycin but to other related antibiotics."[6]

Neosporin Topical Ointment was one of the topical antibiotics reviewed by the NAS-NRC as part of the drug efficacy program. It and the other topical antibiotics were rated less-than-effective for use in a variety of skin problems. These products are promoted and prescribed for minor wound healing, for skin infections such as impetigo and for the prevention of infections following minor cuts, burns and abrasions. Neosporin Topical has also been used in the treatment of skin ulcers and infected eczemas.

Topical antibiotic products containing neomycin have also been examined by an FDA advisory panel on OTC drugs.[7] It declared that over-the-counter skin application products containing neomycin lack satisfactory evidence of effectiveness for any medical purpose. Although further studies are pending, the products cannot presently be recognized as clinically satisfactory. Other reports support this conclusion.[8]

Besides the disadvantages mentioned, there can be dangerous side effects. Taken by injection or by pill, neomycin has been known to cause hearing loss and kidney damage. These routes of administration surely involve larger blood stream exposure to neomycin than that which is absorbed via the skin. As the FDA has stated, it is not even known what amount of neomycin enters the blood stream from the skin in either the proper use or the potential misuses of the drug. Furthermore, it is not known what amount of neomycin is small enough to not cause adverse reactions. Until these two facts are known, it must be assumed that skin exposure to neomycin also presents some risk of deafness and kidney damage, especially if the skin is broken (which would enhance absorption). In our view, the rare but potentially serious adverse effects of neomycin in skin products makes it unacceptable, particularly because it has not been proven effective in such products.

Even though the law requires controlled proof of effectiveness, the FDA permits continued marketing of these products. Since some are available OTC as well as by prescription, it is difficult to say just how often they are used by the public. Nevertheless, the drug Neosporin, probably the most popular of these preparations and available in cream, ointment and powder, filled 1,350,000 prescriptions in 1979. This figure is undoubtedly only a fraction of its total sales since it does not include OTC business.

As part of its comprehensive OTC drug review, the FDA has proposed putting these products of unproven effectiveness and/or safety in a so-called "Category III" classification which a Federal Court has found illegal.[9] In the case of these neomycin-containing OTC products, they remain of unproven safety and efficacy. Manufacturers have known since 1962 that proof of effectiveness is required by law but have not generated such proof in the intervening 19 years.

Given the mandates of the 1962 Drug Law (see History), the topical antibiotic preparations cited in this guide should be removed immediately from the market until or unless they are proven safe and effective. Even in the context of the American OTC drug market, which has been aptly described as a jungle of "rip-offs,"[10] these skin antibiotics strike us as outstandingly bad products.

Steroid Antibiotic Combinations

There are some 60 drugs of unproven effectiveness for skin, eye or ear application mentioned in this guide that are ointments, creams and lotions containing an *adrenal corticosteroid* (cortisone-like) agent in combination with *antibacterial* and/or *antifungal* drugs. In 25 of the products, neomycin is combined with steroids. By and large, they are promoted for wound healing, for the resolution of skin infections of bacterial and/or fungal origin, for the prevention of infections secondary to burns and for the treatment of skin inflammation where bacterial infection is possible. The addition of antibiotic agents such as neomycin, *nystatin* and *gramicidin* to corticosteroids may seem logical, but there is insufficient evidence of efficacy for any of these topical combinations.

Although steroids alone may be effective in treating non-infected skin, their use with antibiotics implies the treatment of infection. In this situation, the use of steroids can be dangerous because they impair the body's defense system and increase the chance of developing or worsening skin infection. According to *AMA Drug Evaluations* (third edition, pg. 918):

> In general, glucocorticoids [corticosteroids] are not preferred for the treatment of cutaneous infections, and antibacterial agents should not be used in the prevention or treatment of noninfectious dermatoses. Also, corticosteroids can suppress signs and symptoms even when they do not cure the causal factors. . .

Mycolog, a product of the E.R. Squibb Company, is fairly representative of this diverse group of antibiotic/steroid combination drugs. It combines two antibacterial agents, neomycin and gramicidin, with an antifungal drug nystatin, and a corticosteroid cream, *triamcinolone acetonide.* Although doctors prescribe Mycolog for the relief of infected rash or inflammation and as an adjunct to skin wound therapy, evidence

36

that it truly works is inadequate. But in 1979, 6.3 million prescriptions were filled for Mycolog in the U.S. at a retail cost of 51 million dollars.

When one does actually develop yeast or fungus infections on the skin, an effective single-ingredient antifungal product, such as nystatin or *tolnaftate,* should be used. When fungus infections on the skin are accompanied by inflammation, itching and scaling, the administration of both *hydrocortisone* and an antifungal agent may be appropriate for a few days. However, both drugs should be administered separately in a proper proportion determined by the physician rather than in a standard fixed-combination ratio, which allows no flexibility in dosage and often forces one to use extra, unnecessary active ingredients. This steroid/antibiotic class of drugs fails to meet the FDA's own guidelines for fixed-combinations, in that each component does not contribute to the therapeutic value and effectiveness of the drug for the prescribed uses.

Why have Mycolog and other combinations like it been permitted to remain on the market? A 1972 Court Order stated that a "limited" number of drugs rated less-than-effective could be temporarily "exempted" from the FDA withdrawal procedures, pending completion of further studies, if it were convincingly shown that there was a "compelling medical need" for these drugs. No such claim can be made for topical combinations such as Mycolog. The FDA has asserted that these drugs should be allowed to remain on the pharmacy shelves because "there are no alternatives available other than one which has been approved since 1962, to which resistant organisms have developed frequently."[11]

However, there is precious little to recommend the use of any antibiotics applied to the skin and to superficial wounds. The FDA stated that further study of available information was necessary to determine the effectiveness for specific conditions. Yet it has been over eight years since the FDA made that statement and placed Mycolog and the others under "exemption." Thus far, there have been no subsequent clarifications of efficacy or proper usage.

After issuing its August 1, 1980 computer printout classifying drugs as effective and not effective, the FDA announced it was going to upgrade 15 drug products from "lacking substantial evidence of effectiveness" to "effective."[12] The 15 products are all ophthalmic (eye) drugs which are combinations of antibiotics and steroids. However, FDA officials have admitted that no studies have been submitted to prove the effectiveness of these products. They have also stated that the main reason for upgrading the drugs to "effective" was heavy pressure from eye doctors. The FDA's approval of these drugs is also inconsistent with the findings of the American Medical Association, which has concluded that these drugs are "irrational mixtures" and that they "are not recommended for the topical [local] treatment of ocular infections."[13]

The dangers of these drugs are discussed in their individual entries in this book. We continue to believe that these drugs are ineffective and dangerous and we strongly recommend against using them; in addition, we are initiating legal action against FDA to challenge its illegal decision upgrading these products to "effective." The fifteen drug products are: Ak-Neo-Cort, Chloromycetin-HC, Cor-Oticin, Cortisporin Ophthalmic Suspension, Metimyd, Neo-Cortef Ophthalmic, Neo-Decadron, Neo-Delta-Cortef Ophthalmic, Neo-Hydeltrasol Ophthalmic, Neo-Medrol Ophthalmic, Neosone, Ophtha P/S Ophthalmic Drops, Ophthel Ointment (Improved), Terra Cortril Ophthalmic, Vasocidin.

FOOTNOTES

[1] North American Contact Dermatitis Group. *Archives of Dermatology.* 108:537, 1973.
[2] Patrick J, Panzer JD. *Archives of Dermatology.* 102:532, 1970.
[3] Epstein E. *JAMA.* 198:517, 1966.
[4] Neomycin is rarely used to treat serious infection now because of its toxicity (although oral neomycin is used in the treatment of hepatic encephalopathy).
[5] *Federal Register.* 42:17661-3.
[6] *Ibid.,* 17661.
[7] Initiated in 1972, this review was designed to achieve what the NAS-NRC review and subsequent Drug Efficacy Study Implementation Project tried to do for the pre-1962 prescription medicines. For a variety of reasons, however, this effort has been characterized by even less progress than the Drug Efficacy Study Implementation Project. An estimated 60 percent of the ingredients in OTC drugs fail to meet safety and effectiveness requirements as mandated by law. *Federal Register.* 37:12857, June 29, 1972.
[8] Davis CM et al. *JAMA.* 203:298, 1968.
[9] The use of "Category III" classification was ruled in violation of the federal Food, Drug and Cosmetic Act by Judge John Sirica in a suit brought by Public Citizen Health Research Group against the Food and Drug Administration. The ruling was made on July 14, 1979.
[10] Graedon J. *The People's Pharmacy.* St. Martin's Press, N.Y., 1976.
[11] *Federal Register.* 37:26624-5, December 14, 1972.
[12] *Federal Register.* 45: 57776, August 29, 1980.
[13] *AMA Drug Evaluation* (first edition, pg. 526), 1971.

PART III: 607 INEFFECTIVE DRUGS

HOW TO USE THIS SECTION

Let's take a hypothetical example in which you visit the doctor complaining of a mild headache and pain of the lower back. After examining you, listening to your story and making the correct diagnosis, the doctor writes on a prescription pad the name *Equagesic,* explaining that it will do the trick for muscular back pain associated with anxiety. Based on the fact that almost 3 million prescriptions for this brand name product were filled in 1979, one can imagine that this happens quite frequently. However, the fact of the matter is that the drug is not effective as a fixed-combination.

Before asking your pharmacist to fill the prescription for Equagesic (costing about $9.00 per fifty pills), you check the index beginning on page xi which tells you that Equagesic is listed on page 98. If your doctor had prescribed *Meprogesic*—which is identical to Equagesic—the index listing for Meprogesic will say "see Equagesic, pg. 98." On that page, you find the brand name, Equagesic; the manufacturer, Wyeth; the use, relief of pain and anxiety; the dosage form, tablet; and the route of administration, oral.

39

1 **Brand Name: EQUAGESIC**
Manufacturer: Wyeth
2 **Use:** Pain relief and anxiety
3 **Dosage Form:** Tablet
4 **Administration:** Oral
5 **Ingredients:** Meprobamate 150 mg (tranquilizer); ethoheptazine citrate 75 mg (analgesic); acetylsalicylic acid 250 mg (analgesic/antipyretic).

6 **EQUAGESIC** is used primarily for the treatment of pain accompanied by tension and/or anxiety in patients with musculoskeletal disease or tension headache.

In the treatment of muscle pain, a hot bath and 2 aspirin tablets will be at least as effective an analgesic (pain reliever) as Equagesic. According to the *AMA Drug Evaluations* (first edition, pg. 186), Equagesic is an "irrational mixture," the "analgesic effect of ethoheptazine is questionable, and there is no conclusive evidence that meprobamate enhances analgesic effectiveness of aspirin alone." Identical drugs include: Meprogesic.

7 **WARNING:** The use of minor tranquilizers such as meprobamate (Miltown), chlordiazepoxide (Librium), diazepam (Valium) or similar drugs during pregnancy should be avoided because of increased risk of damage to the developing fetus. One must consider the possibility of pregnancy when beginning minor tranquilizer therapy. In the case of combination drugs such as Equagesic, use at any time is unwarranted.

Next we see there are three ingredients: a mild tranquilizer *meproba-mate* and two analgesics (pain relievers), *ethoheptazine* and *acetyl-salicylic acid* (aspirin). Indications for Equagesic are for the treatment of pain accompanied by tension and/or anxiety in patients with musculo-skeletal disease or tension headache.

1. ***Brand Name*** (or generic name if only one ingredient) and ***Manufac-turer***

   Because two-thirds of the less-than-effective products cited in this book contain more than one ingredient in a fixed-combination, most of the headings are brand names. Prescription drugs are usually sold in more than one strength and may have several different dosage forms (e.g., tablet, capsule, syrup). Some of the products included in this book come in as many as nine different strengths or dosage forms. A few drug manufacturers reflect this fact by adding letters and/or numbers to the brand name, although most do not. For example, *Milpath 200* and *Milpath 400* refer to the amount of the tranquilizer component (in milligrams) included in each tablet form. Other companies differentiate the strengths of the same drug by using phrases such as "forte" (stronger) or "lontabs" (time-release) in the names. All brand names are capitalized.

2. ***Use***

   The general purpose (indication) for the drug is described, such as "cough and cold," "digestive disorders" or "pain relief." This is not meant to list all of the possible reasons why doctors prescribe this drug, but is useful in categorizing its general function.

3. ***Dosage Form***

   Capsules, Cream, Drops and Syrup are examples of dosage forms, in other words, how the drug is supplied.

4. ***Administration***

   This heading explains how the drug product is brought into contact with your body. This can make a great difference in the safety and ef-fectiveness of the drug. For example, some drugs, such as *Proternol,* are rated effective if they are injected into a vein, but are considered less-than-effective when given orally, because during the absorption process and passage through the liver, the drug is broken down to an inactive form. Therefore, it is important to understand how the drugs you use enter and affect your system. To avoid confusion, we have made distinctions, when appropriate, between different forms of the same drug by explicitly including the route of administration in the brand name heading, for example *Neo-Decadron Topical.* Other examples of route of administration include: Intravenous, Intra-muscular and Eye.

5. *Ingredients*

The common or generic name for each ingredient is listed. When it is considered helpful, the actual amount (in milligrams) of each ingredient is cited after each generic name. Next to each ingredient in parentheses is listed the basic action of each: "sedative," "anticholinergic," "vasodilator" (see glossary for explanation of these terms).

6. The diseases or diagnoses for which these ineffective drugs are most often promoted or prescribed are described here. Most of the uses cited are based on the official FDA-approved drug labeling. Many drugs are also used for medical problems for which the FDA has not given approval. In some cases, we have included these as well. The rest of the text explains further why a hot bath and two aspirins would be as effective as Equagesic, probably safer, and would save quite a bit of money. Finally, drugs with active ingredients that are identical to Equagesic are also included.

7. *Warnings*

All drugs have side effects or dangers; but if they are effective, the benefits can outweigh the risks. For all 607 drugs listed in this book, evidence of effectiveness is lacking, so whatever the risks are, they, by definition, outweigh the benefits and we do not recommend using the drugs. Box warnings that appear in the official labeling of any of these drugs are always included.

Most of the drugs in Part III fall into one of the five following categories. The entries for these drugs will refer you to the case studies on these categories, for a more detailed discussion. These five, in Part II, "Treatment for Common Diseases," are:

1. Drugs for Cough, Cold and Allergy
2. Drugs for Heart Pain
3. Drugs for Circulatory Disorders of Head and Limbs
4. Drugs for Digestive Disorders
5. Drugs Applied Directly to Skin, Eye or Ear.

Finally, Part III includes a number of drugs which are not in any of these five categories. These may be single drug entries or narrow groups of drugs. In the case of these smaller groups, you may be referred to the drug of that small category that contains the most extensive information.

- **Brand Name: ACHROSTATIN-V**
- **Manufacturer:** Lederle
- **Use:** Infection
- **Dosage Form:** Capsule
- **Administration:** Oral
- **Ingredients:** Tetracycline hydrochloride 250 mg (antibacterial); nystatin 250,000 units (antifungal).

ACHROSTATIN-V is a fixed-combination product promoted for infections of bacterial and fungal origin. According to the *AMA Drug Evaluations* (third edition, p. 752), it is preferable to prescribe nystatin, a useful antifungal agent, on an individual basis if combined therapy with a broad spectrum antibiotic is considered desirable. By prescribing it separately, if needed, your doctor can better determine the proper amount for your medical problem. The amount of nystatin included in Achrostatin-V is insufficient to cope with most fungal infections. Nystatin can cause nausea and vomiting. Identical drugs include: Tetrastatin.

See similar drug MYSTECLIN F, pg. 122

- **Brand Name: ACTIFED**
- **Manufacturer:** Burroughs Wellcome
- **Use:** Cold and allergy
- **Dosage Form:** Syrup / Tablet
- **Administration:** Oral / Oral
- **Ingredients:** Triprolidine hydrochloride (antihistamine); pseudoephedrine hydrochloride (sympathomimetic).

ACTIFED is promoted and used for treatment of hay fever and common cold symptoms. Triprolidine is an effective antihistamine for the relief of hay fever and other allergic conditions, but there is no satisfactory evidence that the so-called "vasoconstrictor" decongestant, pseudoephedrine, enhances the effects of antihistamines in the allergy patient. For allergy, antihistamines alone are most appropriate. Pseudoephedrine can cause or aggravate high blood pressure and commonly loses its effectiveness when used regularly, while triprolidine can cause drowsiness, loss of coordination, mental inattention and dizziness. Identical drugs include: Actacin, Actagen, Actamine, Allerfrin, Allerphed, Dri-Phed, Eldafed, Eldefed, Norafed, Pseudo-Prol, Sudahist, Tagafed, Tri-Fed, Triafed, Triphed, Triprolidine HCl with Pseudoephedrine HCl.

Also see Part II: Drugs for Cough, Cold and Allergy

- **Brand Name: ACTIFED-C EXPECTORANT**
- **Manufacturer:** Burroughs Wellcome
- **Use:** Cough, cold, allergy
- **Dosage Form:** Syrup
- **Administration:** Oral
- **Ingredients:** Codeine phosphate 10 mg (antitussive/narcotic); triprolidine hydrochloride 2 mg (antihistamine); pseudoephedrine hydrochloride 30 mg (sympathomimetic); guaifenesin 100 mg (expectorant) per 5 ml.

ACTIFED-C EXPECTORANT has been found by the FDA to lack substantial evidence of effectiveness as a fixed-combination for the symptomatic relief of cough in conditions such as the common cold, acute bronchitis, allergic asthma, croup and emphysema. This is a blatant example of an ineffective, irrational fixed-dosage cough and cold combination product. Only one of the individual ingredients, codeine, is of genuine therapeutic value in treating cough symptoms. However, patients with dry, hacking cough should instead use dextromethorphan. The antihistamine triprolidine has no proven effectiveness in treating either cough or the common cold. Guaifenesin is an expectorant of highly dubious value in relieving coughs.

The NAS-NRC had good reason to rate Actifed-C "ineffective" as a fixed-combination and consumers should stay away from it and similar mixtures. It is disturbing that doctors continue to prescribe such products with great frequency. Codeine often causes drowsiness and constipation and is psychologically and physically addicting when taken regularly. Pseudoephedrine can cause or aggravate high blood pressure and commonly loses its effectiveness when used regularly. Triprolidine can cause drowsiness, loss of coordination, mental inattention and dizziness. Identical drugs include: Actacin-C, Allerphed C Expectorant, Cophed-C Expectorant, Dri-Phed w/ Codeine Expectorant.

Also see Part II: Drugs for Cough, Cold and Allergy

- **Brand Name: ADRENOSEM SALICYLATE**
- **Manufacturer:** Beecham
- **Use:** Bleeding
- **Dosage Form:** Syrup / Tablet / Solution
- **Administration:** Oral / Oral / Intramuscular
- **Ingredients:** Carbazochrome salicylate (coagulant).

ADRENOSEM SALICYLATE is used to

control various surgical and other bleeding states. The FDA has reported that there are no adequate and well-controlled clinical studies conducted by scientific experts to demonstrate the effectiveness of the drug. It has been found "ineffective" for all uses recommended in the labeling.

- Brand Name: **ADROYD**
- **Manufacturer:** Parke-Davis
- **Use:** Bone, growth disorders
- **Dosage Form:** Tablet
- **Administration:** Oral
- **Ingredients:** Oxymetholone 5 or 10 mg (androgenic steroid).

ADROYD (a weak male hormone), is marketed for use as supportive therapy in the treatment of senile and postmenopausal bone disorders (progressive decrease in total bone mass). It has been used in children for the management of certain growth disorders, but this may result in irreversible adverse effects. The National Academy of Sciences-National Research Council cautions that the use of these hormones in the treatment of progressive bone disorder (osteoporosis) is without value as a primary therapy. Its side effects can include masculinization of women. The current labeling for this drug stresses that for bone disorders equal or greater consideration should be given to diet, calcium balance, physical therapy and good health-promoting measures.

See similar drug WINSTROL, pg. 188

- Brand Name: **AEROSPORIN OTIC SOLUTION**
- **Manufacturer:** Burroughs Wellcome
- **Use:** Ear infection
- **Dosage Form:** Solution
- **Administration:** Ear
- **Ingredients:** Polymyxin B sulfate 10,000 u (antibacterial) per ml.

AEROSPORIN OTIC SOLUTION is

promoted for the treatment of external ear infections caused by certain groups of bacteria. The FDA has determined that it is in-effective for such treatment. When used topically in the ear, antibacterial agents can produce sensitivity reactions. For serious external ear infections, oral antibiotics are appropriate. However, a culture should always be taken to determine first what organism is causing the infection.

Also see Part II: Drugs Applied Directly to Skin, Eye or Ear

- Brand Name: **ALEVAIRE**
- **Manufacturer:** Breon
- **Use:** Asthma, respiratory disorders
- **Dosage Form:** Solution
- **Administration:** Inhale
- **Ingredients:** Tyloxapol 0.125% (detergent); glycerin 5%; sodium bicarbonate 2%.

ALEVAIRE, a detergent solution, is used to lower surface tension in the lungs and help liquify mucus. It is promoted and prescribed for the short-term management of many inflammatory and post-operative lung conditions. Sometimes it is administered inter-mittently in the long-term management of certain chronic pulmonary (lung) diseases, such as cystic fibrosis. There is no substantial clinical evidence that Alevaire is any more effective than an aerosol solution of sodium chloride (table salt) or pure water, and further-more, prolonged use of tyloxapol may irritate the lungs.

- Brand Name: **AMBENYL EXPECTORANT**
- **Manufacturer:** Marion
- **Use:** Cough and cold
- **Dosage Form:** Syrup
- **Administration:** Oral
- **Ingredients:** Codeine sulfate 10 mg (antitussive/narcotic); bromodiphenhydramine hydrochloride 3.75 mg, diphenhydramine hydrochloride 8.75 mg (antihistamines); guaiacolsulfonate potas-sium 80 mg, ammonium chloride 80 mg (expectorants) per 5 ml, alcohol 5%.

AMBENYL EXPECTORANT is a fixed-combination drug which has been rated ineffective by the FDA. Why two antihistamines, whose effect is to dry up secretions, are combined with two drugs supposed to loosen secretions, is hard to imagine. Reputable medical literature does not support the use of this irrational mixture nor ones like it. Ammonium chloride can be harmful to patients with improperly functioning lungs, liver, or kidneys while bromodiphenhydramine and diphenhydramine can cause drowsiness, loss of coordination, mental inattention and dizziness. Identical drugs include: Bromanyl Expectorant.

See similar drug PHENERGAN EXPECTORANT, pg. 157 Also see Part II: Drugs for Cough, Cold and Allergy

- **Brand Name: AMESEC**
- **Manufacturer:** Lilly
- **Use:** Asthma, respiratory disorders
- **Dosage Form:** Tablet /Capsule
- **Administration:** Oral / Oral
- **Ingredients:** Aminophylline 130 mg, ephedrine hydrochloride 25 mg (bronchodilators); amobarbital 25 mg (sedative).

AMESEC is a fixed-combination drug product prescribed for the prevention and symptomatic treatment of asthma and related respiratory problems. One of the ingredients, aminophylline, is an important drug used primarily to treat mild asthma and asthma-like symptoms associated with certain respiratory conditions such as bronchitis; its dosage in Amesec is much smaller than the usual adult dose. Ephedrine, an adrenalin-like drug, dilates air passages and is used in treating asthma; however, it may cause or aggravate high blood pressure. In addition, ephedrine often loses its effectiveness when given on a prolonged basis.

The efficacy of barbiturates, such as amobarbital, in the treatment of asthma is not proven; they may suppress the breathing impulse, and worsen severe asthma. Single-drug asthma products, such as aminophylline or theophylline, will often prevent or control bronchospasm; fixed-ratio combinations are unnecessary. Moreover, many of the fixed combinations such as Amesec do not contain adequate amounts of the effective single ingredients to justify their use. When taken regularly amobarbital can lead to psychological and physical addiction. Identical drugs include: Amo-Fed, Amphed.

- **Brand Name: AMINOBRAIN PT**
- **Manufacturer:** Panamericana
- **Use:** Central nervous system stimulation
- **Dosage Form:** Elixir
- **Administration:** Oral
- **Ingredients:** Pentylenetetrazol 100 mg (stimulant/analeptic); niacin 50 mg (vitamin/vasodilator); lysine hydrochloride 100 mg (amino acid); vitamin B-1 1 mg, B-2 1.2 mg (vitamins), alcohol 5%.

AMINOBRAIN PT is a combination drug comprised of a central nervous system (CNS) stimulant and a number of vitamins (one with vessel dilating properties). It is recommended by the manufacturer to enhance the mental and physical activity of elderly patients. There is no evidence to support the manufacturer's claims and this product has no place in proper medical care.

See similar drug RU-VERT, pg. 172

- **Brand Name: AMINOPHYLLINE AND AMYTAL**
- **Manufacturer:** Lilly
- **Use:** Asthma, respiratory disorders
- **Dosage Form:** Tablet
- **Administration:** Oral
- **Ingredients:** Aminophylline 100 mg (bronchodilator); amobarbital 32 mg (sedative).

AMINOPHYLLINE AND AMYTAL is a fixed-ratio mixture sold for the prevention and symptomatic treatment of asthma and related breathing problems. It is very similar to another Eli Lilly drug product, Amesec, except that it does not include the ingredient ephedrine hydrochloride. Aminophylline can be effective for treating asthma if used at the proper individualized dose. The dose in this product may not be effective for many people. This product also contains amobarbital (a barbiturate) for which there is no clinical evidence of effectiveness in the treatment of asthma and which can lead to psychological and physical addiction if used regularly.

See similar drug AMESEC, pg. 47

- **Brand Name: AMODRINE**
- **Manufacturer:** Searle
- **Use:** Asthma, respiratory disorders
- **Dosage Form:** Tablet
- **Administration:** Oral
- **Ingredients:** Aminophylline 100 mg, racephedrine hydrochloride 25 mg (bronchodilators); phenobarbital 8 mg (sedative).

AMODRINE is used in the treatment of respiratory disorders involving bronchospasms and asthma. This fixed-combination drug contains the sedative phenobarbital (a barbiturate) for which there is no clinical evidence to demonstrate its effectiveness in the treatment of asthma. The use of fixed-ratio combinations as a substitute for single-drug preparations of aminophylline or theophylline is unnecessary. Aminophylline can be effective for treating asthma if used at the proper individualized dose. The dose in Amodrine may not be effective for many people.

The small amount of racephedrine, a stimulant, may aggravate high blood pressure in the hypertensive patient. When taken regularly phenobarbital can lead to psychological and physical addiction.

See similar drug AMESEC, pg. 47

- **Brand Name: ANANASE-50, -100**
- **Manufacturer:** Rorer
- **Use:** Inflammation
- **Dosage Form:** Enteric coated tablet
- **Administration:** Oral
- **Ingredients:** Bromelains 50,000 or 100,000 u (anti-inflammatory enzyme).

ANANASE is promoted as supportive therapy for the reduction of inflammation and the excessive accumulation of fluid in the tissue spaces (edema). It is also used to ease pain, speed healing and accelerate tissue repair. The FDA has, rated Ananase as ineffective for its prescribed uses.

- **Brand Name: ANTORA-B T.D.**
- **Manufacturer:** Mayrand
- **Use:** Heart pain (angina pectoris)
- **Dosage Form:** Time-release capsule
- **Administration:** Oral
- **Ingredients:** Pentaerythritol tetranitrate 30 mg (coronary vaso-dilator); secobarbital 50 mg (sedative).

ANTORA-B is administered to prevent, control and treat transient pain of coronary artery disease (angina pectoris). It is usually prescribed when the physician believes that anxiety or emotional disturbances may be important factors. However, there is no convincing evidence that pentaerythritol tetranitrate is of value in the long-term management of angina. Nor is there persuasive clinical evidence to support this particular fixed-ratio combination.

Pentaerythritol tetranitrate is a coronary vasodilator with definite effects on blood flow. However, it has not been proven effective in reducing the severity or frequency of anginal attacks. Furthermore, there is no satisfactory evidence that the regular use of a sedative in such a combined product confers significant therapeutic benefit. If occasional anxiety in the angina patient is a real problem, a sedative, adjusted to the specific needs of the patient, and nitroglycerin (sublingual) should be administered separately. Daily use of barbiturates is not wise, since physical and psychological addiction can result. Identical drugs include: Corovas Tymcaps.

Also see Part II: Drugs for Heart Pain

- **Brand Name: ARLIDIN**
- **Manufacturer:** USV
- **Use:** Blood vessel disease (head and limbs)
- **Dosage Form:** Tablet
- **Administration:** Oral
- **Ingredients:** Nylidrin hydrochloride 6 or 12 mg (vasodilator).

ARLIDIN is promoted for use in controlling the symptoms of vasospastic (vessel "constriction") peripheral vascular disorders, such as cramp-like pains and weakness in the legs, cold hands and feet and vertigo. It is also used in circulatory disturbances of the inner ear. However, there is no convincing evidence that Arlidin is of therapeutic value in the treatment of the above disorders or other conditions for which it has been promoted (such as cerebrovascular disorders). Currently, there are no drugs rated effective for symptoms due to obstructive peripheral blood vessel diseases. Identical drugs include: Nylidrin HC1.

Also see Part II: Drugs for Circulatory Disorders of Head and Limbs

- **Brand Name: ASMINYL**
- **Manufacturer:** O'Neal, Jones and Feldman
- **Use:** Asthma, respiratory disorders
- **Dosage Form:** Tablet
- **Administration:** Oral
- **Ingredients:** Theophylline 130 mg, ephedrine sulfate 32 mg (bronchodilators); sodium phenobarbital 8 mg (sedative).

ASMINYL is a combination product used in the symptomatic treatment of asthma and other respiratory disorders. However, no substantial clinical evidence exists to demonstrate the effectiveness of such a combination product.

The sedative phenobarbital has no proven effect in the treatment of asthmatic conditions. Phenobarbital is included in these combinations supposedly to counteract the central stimulation effects caused by theophylline and ephedrine. The amount of phenobarbital present is too small to have any measurable sedative effect. All bronchodilator sedative combinations lack the necessary evidence to qualify as effective for long-term prevention and treatment of asthmatic attacks and other respiratory problems.

Single-entity drugs, such as aminophylline or theophylline, will usually control acute attacks of bronchospasm. These drugs usually are among the active ingredient(s) of fixed-combination products, such as Asminyl, but are easily available alone in oral generic form. If a sedative is needed to counteract the effects of a bronchodilating agent, then it should be administered separately at a dosage adjusted to specific needs. Most people do perfectly well with a single bronchodilator and should avoid fixed-combinations that expose them to unnecessary drugs and thereby increase the risk of unwanted side effects and drug interactions. The 32 mg of ephedrine, a stimulant, included in Asminyl may aggravate high blood pressure in the patient with hypertension. When taken regularly, phenobarbital can lead to psychological and physical addiction.

- **Brand Name: ATARAXOID**
- **Manufacturer:** Pfizer
- **Use:** Inflammation, allergy
- **Dosage Form:** Tablet
- **Administration:** Oral
- **Ingredients:** Prednisolone 2.5 or 5 mg (corticosteroid); hydroxyzine hydrochloride 10 mg (antihistamine/tranquilizer).

ATARAXOID is used for the symptomatic relief of inflammation (swelling, redness, heat and pain) and itching resulting from a number of types of allergies and other disorders. The FDA has rated the product as ineffective. In general, the use of fixed-combinations containing adrenal corticosteroid hormones is discouraged. Prolonged use or excessive dosage can impair the body's defense mechanisms against infectious disease. Ataraxoid also contains hydroxyzine, a drug with both tranquilizing and antihistaminic properties. Although drugs such as prednisolone alone may be effective for short-term therapy of self-limited allergic conditions, the use of the combination drug Ataraxoid is inappropriate. Hydroxyzine can cause drowsiness, loss of coordination, mental inattention and dizziness.

- **Brand Name: AVAZYME**
- **Manufacturer:** Wallace
- **Use:** Inflammation
- **Dosage Form:** Enteric coated tablet
- **Administration:** Oral
- **Ingredients:** Crystalline chymotrypsin 20 or 40 mg (anti-inflammatory enzyme).

AVAZYME is promoted for the relief of symptoms related to certain obstetrical procedures (episiotomy) and also as adjunctive therapy in the treatment of inflammation and tissue swelling resulting from serious surgical or accidental trauma. However, the FDA has rated Avazyme as ineffective for these clinical uses. Identical drugs include: Avazyme-100.

- **Brand Name: AVC CREAM**
- **Manufacturer:** Merrell-National
- **Use:** Vaginal infection
- **Dosage Form:** Cream
- **Administration:** Vaginal
- **Ingredients:** Sulfanilamide 15%, allantoin 2%, aminacrine hydrochloride 0.2% (anti-infectives).

AVC CREAM is used for the relief of symptoms of vaginal infection when the specific organism responsible is not known. Recently, two FDA scientific advisory groups recommended that the three AVC products (Cream, Suppositories, Dienestrol), along with 112 related vaginal sulfa preparations, be removed from the market because they are ineffective. Only selected products are listed in this guide.

Manufacturers claim that AVC products should be used for vaginitis where diagnosis is supposedly impossible. Yet most experts shun the "shotgun" approach to vaginal infections implied by the AVC drug ads. In *Medical Word News*,[1] Dr. Raymond Kaufman, head of obstetrics-gynecology at Baylor Medical College in Houston, asserts that "careful diagnosis has shown that for more than 90% of patients with nonspecific vaginitis, the cause is Hemophilus vaginalis [a type of bacteria]." Yet it has been found that vaginal infections caused by this organism persist in some 86% of women treated with a sulfanilamide cream such as AVC.

The *AMA Drug Evaluations* (first edition, pg. 471) calls AVC "an irrational mixture of sulfanilamide, aminacrine and allantoin." There is no conclusive evidence that aminacrine hydrochloride is effective against the bacteria and yeasts that usually cause vaginal infections. Moreover, the topical use of the antibiotic sulfanilamide is inefficacious and poor medical practice. The *AMA Drug Evaluations* (second edition, pg. 555) states that "topically applied sulfonamides [such as sulfanilamide] are generally ineffective in the management of infections in wounds and infections of the skin and mucus membrane, possibly because pus and cellular debris inhibit their action. They also have a greater tendency to produce sensitization [allergic reaction], which can preclude their later systemic [oral] administration."

Doctors are turning increasingly to orally-administered antibiotics to treat vaginal infections when the causative organism(s) has been clearly identified by culture. However, because some physicians believe that these oral antibiotics should be used only for more serious diseases, they recommend that before taking medication patients try simple measures, such as wearing cotton underwear and using mildly acidic douches.

The most common side effects of AVC products are allergic reactions, such as rashes, local itching, burning sensation and fever. Although the amount of sulfanilamide usually absorbed with normal AVC use is unlikely to produce major sulfonamide toxicity, there is a risk involved. Sulfonamides are potent antibiotics with serious potential adverse reactions. They are known to produce rare, sometimes fatal, disorders of the blood that are indicated by easy bruising, delayed clotting, cuts that don't heal, sore throat and fever.

According to Dr. King Holmes, Associate Professor of Medicine at the University of Washington and Chief of Infectious Diseases at the U.S. Public Health Service Hospital in Seattle,[2] surveys estimate that manufacturers earn some $50 million annually on the sale of topical sulfa vaginal preparations. As reported in *Medical World News,* he calls it the "$50 million rip-off." Identical drugs include: Amide-VC Cream, Cervex Cream, Deltavac Cream, Femguard Cream, Par Cream, Sufamal Cream, Tricholan Cream, Triconol Cream, Vagacreme, Vag Cream, Vagidine Cream, Vagimine Cream, Vagi-Nil Cream, Vagitrol Cream.

[1] *Medical World News* 20:16, 35, August 6, 1979.
[2] *Ibid.*

- Brand Name: **AVC/DIENESTROL CREAM**
- **Manufacturer:** Merrell-National
- **Use:** Vaginal infection
- **Dosage Form:** Cream
- **Administration:** Vaginal
- **Ingredients:** Dienestrol 0.01% (estrogen); sulfanilamide 15%, allantoin 2%, aminacrine hydrochloride 0.2% (anti-infectives).

AVC/DIENESTROL CREAM is an estrogen-containing mixture prescribed for the treatment of several vaginal infections characterized by atrophy (thinning of vaginal lining) and complicated by bacterial or yeast infection. The FDA has rated AVC Dienestrol as less than effective as a combination product, based on the review of AVC Cream and Suppositories by the NAS-NRC scientific panel. Furthermore, there is substantial clinical evidence that estrogens increase the risk of developing cancer of the uterus (womb) in post-menopausal women. Dienestrol has been shown to be significantly absorbed through the vagina. Sulfanilamide, another ingredient in AVC Dienestrol, can cause allergic reactions such as rashes and, more rarely, serious blood disorders.

See similar drug AVC CREAM, pg. 53

- Brand Name: **AVC SUPPOSITORIES**
- **Manufacturer:** Merrell-National
- **Use:** Vaginal infection
- **Dosage Form:** Suppository
- **Administration:** Vaginal
- **Ingredients:** Sulfanilamide 1.05 gm, allantoin 0.14 gm, aminacrine hydrochloride .014 gm (anti-infectives).

AVC SUPPOSITORIES are promoted and prescribed for the relief of symptoms of vaginal infections where the isolation of the specific organism causing the infection is not possible. There is insufficient evidence of clinical efficacy to justify their use. Sulfanilamide can cause allergic reactions such as rashes, and, more rarely, serious blood disorders. Identical drugs include: Par-Vag Suppositories, Tricholan Suppositories, Triconol Suppositories, Vagitrol Suppositories, Vasucap Suppositories.

See similar drug AVC CREAM, pg. 53

See similar drug AVC CREAM, pg. 53

- Brand Name: **AZO GANTANOL**
- **Manufacturer:** Roche
- **Use:** Urinary tract infection
- **Dosage Form:** Tablet
- **Administration:** Oral
- **Ingredients:** Sulfamethoxazole 500 mg (antibacterial); phenazopyridine hydrochloride 100 mg (urinary tract analgesic).

AZO GANTANOL is prescribed for urinary tract infections complicated by pain. One of the drug's components, phenazopyridine, is said to reduce pain in the urinary tract, but this claim is doubted by many doctors. If pain associated with urinary tract infections is really a problem, the physician should prescribe an analgesic of proven efficacy. Sulfa drugs such as sulfamethoxazole can cause allergic reactions, headache, dizziness, nausea, vomiting, and, rarely, serious blood disorders. Phenazopyridine can cause yellow staining of the skin and should not be used by patients with liver or kidney problems.

See similar drug UROBIOTIC-250, pg. 183

See similar drug UROBIOTIC-250, pg. 183

- **Brand Name: AZOTREX**
- **Manufacturer:** Bristol
- **Use:** Urinary tract infection
- **Dosage Form:** Capsule
- **Administration:** Oral
- **Ingredients:** Tetracycline 125 mg, sulfamethizole 250 mg (antibacterials); phenazopyridine hydrochloride 50 mg (urinary tract analgesic).

AZOTREX is a combination drug promoted for urinary tract infections and accompanying pain in adults. Since no additive action has been demonstrated for the two antibacterial components tetracycline and sulfamethizole, the use of proper doses of either agent alone is preferred. Phenazopyridine is of dubious value as a painkiller and should not be used by patients with liver or kidney disorders. According to the *AMA Drug Evaluations* (first edition, pg. 420), combinations of fixed-ratios of a sulfonamide and another antibacterial, as is found in Azotrex, are "irrational" and "not recommended." There is no substantial evidence that mixed infections requiring combined use of the two antibacterials in Azotrex actually occur. Moreover, combining antibacterials can actually reduce their effectiveness. The recommended dose, 4-8 pills per day, is as little as one half of the accepted therapeutic dose of either antibacterial, meaning that a patient may get inadequate therapy. Also, the use of a combination such as Azotrex subjects the patient to the potential adverse effects of the additional drugs. Sulfa drugs such as sulfamethizole can cause allergic reactions, headache, dizziness, nausea, vomiting and, rarely, serious blood disorders. Phenazopyridine can cause yellow staining of the skin and should not be used by patients with liver or kidney problems.

See similar drug UROBIOTIC-250, pg. 183

- **Brand Name: BACIMYCIN**
- **Manufacturer:** Merrell-National
- **Use:** Skin disorders
- **Dosage Form:** Ointment
- **Administration:** Topical
- **Ingredients:** Neomycin sulfate 5.0 mg, zinc bacitracin 500 u (antibacterials) per gm.

BACIMYCIN, a fixed-combination topical ointment, is prescribed for a variety of skin disorders involving infection or the threat of infection. It is also available without a prescription. Its indications include treatment of biopsy sites, skin ulcers and boils, minor burns, infected eczema and related skin problems, such as impetigo. This preparation is also administered to prevent infection whenever the skin has been broken. Neomycin commonly causes skin rashes and can sensitize people to other more important antibiotics.

Also see Part II: Drugs Applied Directly to Skin, Eye or Ear

- Brand Name: **BARBIDONNA**
- **Manufacturer:** Wallace
- **Use:** Digestive disorders
- **Dosage Form:** Tablet /Elixir
- **Administration:** Oral / Oral
- **Ingredients:** Hyoscyamine sulfate, atropine sulfate and scopolamine (antispasmodics/antisecretories); phenobarbital (sedative); alcohol 15% (in elixir).

BARBIDONNA has virtually the same composition and uses as Donnatal. When taken regularly phenobarbital can lead to psychological and physical addiction. Hyoscyamine, atropine and scopolamine often cause blurring of vision, dryness of the mouth and throat, constipation and hesitancy of urination.

See similar drug DONNATAL, pg. 93
Also see Part II: Drugs for Digestive Disorders

- Brand Name: **BELLADENAL**
- **Manufacturer:** Sandoz
- **Use:** Digestive disorders
- **Dosage Form:** Time-release tablet
- **Administration:** Oral
- **Ingredients:** Belladonna alkaloids 0.25 mg (antispasmodic/ antisecretory); phenobarbital 50 mg (sedative).

BELLADENAL is prescribed as adjunctive therapy in the treatment of stomach ulcer, irritable bowel syndrome and other gastrointestinal disorders. The FDA has stated that it lacks the necessary evidence of efficacy as a fixed-combination for its labeled indications. The *AMA Drug Evaluations* (first edition, pg. 593) states that such mixtures are irrational and are not recommended, because patients requiring large doses of the antispasmodic (belladonna alkaloids) would be bothered by the sedative effect of the other ingredient (phenobarbital).

Fifty milligrams of phenobarbital is a sizeable dose (most drugs of this kind contain 16 mg or 32 mg) and may cause significant drowsiness; it can also cause drug addiction when taken chronically. This kind of rigid formulation is exactly the sort of product that carries with it the disadvantages and liabilities inherent in fixed-ratio combination drugs. When taken regularly, phenobarbital can lead to psychological and physical addiction. Belladonna alkaloids often cause blurring of vision, dryness of the mouth and throat, constipation, and hesitancy of urination. Identical drugs include: Belladenal-S.

Also see Part II: Drugs for Digestive Disorders

- Brand Name: **BENADRYL WITH EPHEDRINE**
- **Manufacturer:** Parke-Davis
- **Use:** Cough, cold, allergy
- **Dosage Form:** Capsule
- **Administration:** Oral
- **Ingredients:** Diphenhydramine hydrochloride 50 mg (antihistamine); ephedrine sulfate 25 mg (sympathomimetic).

BENADRYL WITH EPHEDRINE is used as a treatment for symptoms of cough, common cold and asthma. While advertised as a cough suppressant, Benadryl (diphenhydramine) has no significant effect on the cough reflex. This combination lacks any ingredient of proven effectiveness for suppressing a cough (dextromethorphan is the preferred agent). Moreover, while diphenhydramine alone is useful in treating the annoying consequences of hay fever and other allergies, it is worthless for cough and cold symptoms. Ephedrine can cause or aggravate high blood pressure and commonly loses its effectiveness when used regularly, while diphenhydramine can cause drowsiness, loss of coordination, mental inattention and dizziness.

Also see Part II: Drugs for Cough, Cold and Allergy

- **Brand Name: BENTYL**
- **Manufacturer:** Merrell-National
- **Use:** Digestive disorders
- **Dosage Form:** Capsule / Syrup / Tablet
- **Administration:** Oral / Oral / Oral
- **Ingredients:** Dicyclomine hydrochloride (antispasmodic/ antisecretory).

BENTYL is a drug promoted and prescribed primarily for ulcer patients and those with irritable bowel syndrome. Related to atropine and belladonna in its effects (antispasmodic/antisecretory), this synthetic product can produce side effects including dry mouth, constipation and urination difficulty. Bentyl has no distinct advantages over other, cheaper synthetic antispasmodics or over the basic substances atropine and belladonna. Identical drugs include: Antispas, Bentomine, Dibent, Dicyclomine HCl, Di-Spaz, Nospaz, Or-Tyl, Spastyl.

Also see Part II: Drugs for Digestive Disorders

- **Brand Name: BENTYL W/PHENOBARBITAL**
- **Manufacturer:** Merrell-National
- **Use:** Digestive disorders
- **Dosage Form:** Tablet / Capsule / Syrup
- **Administration:** Oral / Oral / Oral
- **Ingredients:** Dicyclomine hydrochloride (antispasmodic/ antisecretory); phenobarbital (sedative); alcohol 19% (in syrup).

BENTYL W/PHENOBARBITAL is a fixed-ratio combination drug which combines the sedative phenobarbital with the antispasmodic dicyclomine. It is prescribed for patients with peptic ulcer and other gastrointestinal disorders thought to be associated with anxiety and tension. However, because fixed-combinations do not allow for independent adjustment of doses, their use is not recommended.

In addition, the antispasmodic dicyclomine hydrochloride can produce side effects including dry mouth, constipation and urination difficulty. When taken regularly, phenobarbital can lead to psychological and physical addiction. Identical drugs include: Bentomine w/Phenobarbital, Dibent-PB, Spastyl w/Phenobarbital.

Also see Part II: Drugs for Digestive Disorders

- **Brand Name:** # BENYLIN COUGH SYRUP
- **Manufacturer:** Parke-Davis
- **Use:** Cough and cold
- **Dosage Form:** Syrup
- **Administration:** Oral
- **Ingredients:** Diphenhydramine hydrochloride 12.5 mg (antihistamine) per 5 ml; alcohol 5%

BENYLIN COUGH SYRUP is sold for the relief of cough due to cold or allergy. It was recently reformulated by it manufacturer to include only the antihistamine diphenhydramine in an alcohol base. Diphenhydramine is a potent antihistamine agent often used to combat allergic symptoms, but it does not suppress cough. The FDA has rated Benylin ineffective, yet it remains a fairly big seller on the prescription cough remedy market. Patients who suffer from a dry, unproductive cough and seek relief should use a medication with generic dextromethorphan as the single ingredient.

Prior to reformulation, Benylin contained several so-called expectorants and menthol. These products, still found in many of the cough preparations cited in this guide, are of highly questionable effectiveness. Nevertheless, diphenhydramine is ineffective as a cough suppressant and can cause drowsiness, loss of coordination, mental inattention and dizziness.

Benylin has an interesting history. Its manufacturer is currently trying, through a lawsuit, to obtain approval to sell this product without a prescription. For a period, Benylin was available without a prescription, but the FDA recently denied Parke-Davis the right to sell it as such. Final resolution of the matter is pending. Identical drugs include: Benachlor (Improved) Cough Syrup, Diphenadril, Diphenallin Cough Syrup, Diphen-Ex Syrup, Diphenhydramine HCl Cough Syrup, Eldadryl (Revised) Cough Syrup, Noradryl Cough Syrup, Tusstat.

Also see Part II: Drugs for Cough, Cold and Allergy

- **Brand Name: BEROCCA-C**
- **Manufacturer:** Roche
- **Use:** Vitamin deficiency
- **Dosage Form:** Solution
- **Administration:** Injection
- **Ingredients:** Vitamin B complex, vitamin C (vitamins).

BEROCCA-C is used in preventing or treating vitamin deficiencies in certain disease states or post-operative conditions. As currently formulated, the injectable multi-vitamin preparation has been found ineffective by the FDA. The FDA claims that there is a medical need for these vitamin products for various clinical conditions, but the issue involved here is the precise formulation. As it is currently marketed, Berocca-C fails to meet the legal requirements for drug effectiveness.

See similar drug FOLBESYN, pg. 102

- **Brand Name: BEROCCA-C 500**
- **Manufacturer:** Roche
- **Use:** Vitamin deficiency
- **Dosage Form:** Solution
- **Administration:** Injection
- **Ingredients:** Vitamin B complex, vitamin C (vitamins).

BEROCCA-C 500, like Berocca-C, has been sold for preventing or treating vitamin deficiencies in certain disease states or post-operative conditions. Its current formulation was rated as ineffective by the FDA in 1972; over the course of eight years there has not been an adequate reformulation of this preparation. All injectable multi-vitamin preparations available today lack substantial evidence of efficacy. This is not to say that the individual vitamins themselves are ineffective, but that proper guidelines have yet to be developed for products that attempt to include all necessary vitamin supplements in one unit.

See similar drug FOLBESYN, pg. 102

- **Brand Name: BETADINE VAGINAL GEL**
- **Manufacturer:** Purdue Frederick
- **Use:** Vaginal infection
- **Dosage Form:** Gel
- **Administration:** Vaginal
- **Ingredients:** Povidone-iodine (anti-infective).

BETADINE VAGINAL GEL is used for treating various vaginal infections, especially those caused by a particular class of protozoans (trichomonas). In 1974, the FDA notified the manufacturer that it was initiating procedures to remove Betadine Vaginal Gel from the market because it lacked evidence of effectiveness, yet it is still available today. Patients may experience allergic reactions to the iodine in this drug.

- **Brand Name: BIOZYME OINTMENT**
- **Manufacturer:** Armour
- **Use:** Wound infection, inflammation
- **Dosage Form:** Ointment
- **Administration:** Topical
- **Ingredients:** Neomycin palmitate 3.5 mg (antibacterial); trypsin-chymotrypsin 10,000 u (enzyme) per gram

BIOZYME OINTMENT is a combination drug used primarily in the treatment of skin wound infections. The enzyme components are included to promote the removal of dead and foreign material from such wounds. The use of topical (applied on the surface) antibiotics alone for skin wounds and infections is at best debatable. Furthermore, neomycin may cause allergic skin reactions and its use could lead to cross sensitization to some other antibiotics. The use of such enzyme-antibacterial mixtures is not advisable.

Also see Part II: Drugs Applied Directly to Skin, Eye or Ear

- **Brand Name: BLEPHAMIDE LIQUIFILM**
- **Manufacturer:** Allergan
- **Use:** Eye infection, inflammation
- **Dosage Form:** Suspension
- **Administration:** Eye
- **Ingredients:** Sodium sulfacetamide 10% (antibacterial), prednisolone acetate 0.2% (corticosteroid); phenylephrine hydrochloride 0.12% (vasoconstrictor).

BLEPHAMIDE LIQUIFILM is used in the treatment of various infections and inflammatory conditions of the eye and eyelid. It contains a corticosteroid in fixed-dose combination with an antibacterial agent. In general, it is inadvisable to employ these mixtures for the routine treatment of eye infections or inflammatory disorders. The use of corticosteroids for the treatment of eye infections may be dangerous because they can either mask the evidence of infection or cause the spreading of infections.

Also see Part II: Drugs Applied Directly to Skin, Eye or Ear

- **Brand Name: BUTAZOLIDIN ALKA**
- **Manufacturer:** Geigy
- **Use:** Arthritis and gout
- **Dosage Form:** Capsule
- **Administration:** Oral
- **Ingredients:** Phenylbutazone 100 mg (anti-inflammatory); aluminum hydroxide 100 mg, magnesium trisilicate 150 mg (antacids).

BUTAZOLIDIN ALKA is prescribed for gout, various arthritic conditions and "painful shoulder". Phenylbutazone alone (Butazolidin) has both anti-inflammatory and analgesic properties and is effective for certain serious forms of arthritis and acute gout attacks. But it is not the preferred drug for these conditions and should not be used for sprains and other minor inflammations.

Severe side effects, including bleeding peptic ulcers and serious—sometimes fatal—abnormalities of the white and red blood cells, can occur. The drug can cause marked salt and water retention, which can worsen high blood pressure and cause leg swelling, especially when used for longer than ten days.

There is no evidence that the two antacids in this expensive form of phenylbutazone prevent ulcers from developing. The FDA has procrastinated for almost six years in the arrangement of a hearing to resolve the question of their efficacy. Technically, this fixed combination product has been rated as ineffective because the antacid components do nothing to diminish the chances of developing gastrointestinal problems from the phenylbutazone. Identical drugs include: Azolid-A, Phenylbutazone Alka, Phenylbutazone Plus, Phenylzone-A.

WARNING: Butazolidin Alka can cause peptic ulcers and bone marrow disease.

- **Brand Name: BUTIBEL**
- **Manufacturer:** McNeil
- **Use:** Digestive disorders
- **Dosage Form:** Tablet / Elixir
- **Administration:** Oral / Oral
- **Ingredients:** Belladonna extract (antispasmodic/antisecretory); butabarbital sodium (sedative); alcohol 7% (in elixir).

BUTIBEL is a fixed-ratio combination product promoted and prescribed as adjunctive therapy for patients with a variety of gastrointestinal problems, such as irritable bowel syndrome. Butibel contains a sedative, butabarbital sodium, and an antispasmodic drug. Butibel is currently marketed without an approved new drug application, which means it has not been shown to possess substantial evidence of efficacy derived from controlled scientific studies. When taken regularly, butabarbital can lead to psychological and physical addiction. Belladonna extract often causes blurring of vision, dryness of the mouth and throat, constipation and hesitancy of urination.

Also see Part II: Drugs for Digestive Disorders

- **Brand Name: BUTIGETIC**
- **Manufacturer:** McNeil
- **Use:** Pain relief
- **Dosage Form:** Tablet
- **Administration:** Oral
- **Ingredients:** Sodium butabarbital 15 mg (sedative); aceta-minophen 200 mg, phenacetin 150 mg (analgesics); caffeine 30 mg (stimulant).

BUTIGETIC is a polypharmaceutical mixture prescribed for the relief of pain associated with a variety of conditions. Of the four ingredients in this product, acetaminophen is the only analgesic of proven safety and efficacy. The sedative, sodium butabarbital, is claimed to enhance the analgesic effectiveness of this product, providing relief of muscle spasm, or relief from anxiety accompanying pain. However, very few properly controlled studies have shown that patients could benefit from combinations of this sort or have proven that such mixtures do, in fact, provide greater symptomatic benefit than the analgesic (acetaminophen) alone. If a sedative is necessary, it should be administered separately rather than in a fixed-ratio combination.

Furthermore, there is no convincing evidence that the inclusion of phenacetin and caffeine with acetaminophen is more effective than acetaminophen alone. Phenacetin has been linked to kidney damage, and there are a few reports that prolonged use may result in kidney cancer and tumors. (*Science,* 204: 4389, 129-30, 1979.)

Butigetic has been deemed ineffective by the FDA and irrational by the *AMA Drug Evaluations* (first edition, p. 187). When taken regularly butabarbital can lead to psychological and physical addiction.

See similar drug SYNALGOS, pg. 174

- **Brand Name: BUTISERPAZIDE PRESTABS 25, 50**
- **Manufacturer:** McNeil
- **Use:** High blood presssure
- **Dosage Form:** Time-release tablet
- **Administration:** Oral
- **Ingredients:** Butabarbital 30 mg (sedative); hydrochlorothiazide 25 or 50 mg (diuretic); reserpine 0.1 mg (antihypertensive).

BUTISERPAZIDE PRESTABS are used

in the treatment of high blood pressure. The FDA has found this fixed-combination drug lacks substantial evidence of effectiveness for hypertension. The *AMA Drug Evaluations* (second edition, pg. 63) states that mixtures that contain a barbiturate, such as Butiserpazide, have no place in anti-high blood pressure therapy. Barbiturates are not effective in lowering blood pressure except when given in hypnotic (sleep-causing) doses. Barbiturates have a high potential for abuse, and their inclusion in these fixed-combinations presents highly unnecessary risks to the patient for no added benefit. (They are even more dangerous because antihypertensive medicines are taken chronically.) If sedation is necessary for a tense or anxious patient, a drug should be given separately in an individualized dosage. When taken regularly, butabarbital can lead to psychological and physical addiction. Drowsiness, diarrhea, nausea, sedation, fatigue, stomach ulceration, slow heartbeat, nasal congestion, muscle stiffness, nightmares and psychological depression are only some of the more common adverse reactions associated with reserpine. In addition, medical studies have linked reserpine to the development of breast cancer in women.

Although the manufacturer is no longer making Butiserpazide it is still available in some pharmacies.

See similar drug RAUTRAX, pg. 165, for discussion of the potential hazards of reserpine.

- **Brand Name: CALDECORT**
- **Manufacturer:** Pennwalt
- **Use:** Skin disorder
- **Dosage Form:** Ointment
- **Administration:** Topical
- **Ingredients:** Hydrocortisone acetate 1% (corticosteroid); undecylenate calcium 3% (antifungal).

CALDECORT is used to treat a wide range of skin disorders when the doctor believes that both an anti-inflammatory agent and an antifungal agent are needed. Some skin fungal infections represent mixed infections of different types of fungi with each other or with bacteria and may not respond unless treated with a specific agent for each organism. Corticosteroids may be needed to combat some kinds of inflammation. However, in general, corticosteroids, such as hydrocortisone, are not preferred for the treatment of skin infections, states *AMA Drug Evaluations* (first edition, pg. 295). Corticosteroids, if they are absorbed in significant amounts, can suppress signs and symptoms of infection, making conditions appear better when they are not. (The chance of this occurring increases when the skin is broken or burned.)

When diagnosing a skin disorder, your doctor should accurately determine whether it is a bacterial infection, a fungal infection or an allergy. Antifungal alternatives, such as tolnaftate and nystatin, which perform better and are more thoroughly tested than undecylenate, are available. If your doctor finds both an antifungal drug and a corticosteroid are required, he or she should administer them separately, with the corticosteroid given for only four to five days.

Also see Part II: Drugs Applied Directly to Skin, Eye or Ear

- **Brand Name: CANTIL W/PHENOBARBITAL**
- **Manufacturer:** Merrell-National
- **Use:** Digestive disorders
- **Dosage Form:** Tablet
- **Administration:** Oral
- **Ingredients:** Mepenzolate bromide 25 mg (antispasmodic/ antisecretory); phenobarbital 16 mg (sedative).

CANTIL W/PHENOBARBITAL is used as back-up therapy in the treatment of various gastrointestinal (G.I.) disorders. Doctors also prescribe it for supportive therapy in the treatment of intestinal outpouching and inflamed G.I. tract mucous membranes. There is insufficient evidence that the addition of a sedative contributes to the therapeutic value of an antispasmodic/ antisecretory agent. Moreover, antispasmodic/antisecretory drugs have not been shown conclusively to aid in the healing of a peptic ulcer, decrease recurrences or prevent complications. Nor is there any evidence to support their use in cases of intestinal outpouching (diverticulitis) or inflammation of the G.I. mucous membrane lining. When taken regularly phenobarbital can lead to psychological and physical addiction. Mepenzolate often causes blurring of vision, dryness of the mouth and throat, constipation and hesitancy of urination.

Also see Part II: Drugs for Digestive Disorders

- **Brand Name: CARBRITAL KAPSEALS**
- **Manufacturer:** Parke-Davis
- **Use:** Anti-anxiety
- **Dosage Form:** Capsule
- **Administration:** Oral
- **Ingredients:** Pentobarbital sodium 97 mg, carbromal 259 mg (sedative/hypnotics).

CARBRITAL is claimed by the manufacturer to relieve severe daytime anxiety without lowering sensory perception, responsiveness to the environment or alertness below safe levels.* Carbrital is also used to treat insomnia.

The FDA has graded Carbrital ineffective as a fixed-combination product. Carbromal adds nothing to the therapeutic effect of pentobarbital. Moreover, such combinations do not permit the careful adjustment of dosage of each drug which is important when administering two or more drugs with different durations of action.

Drowsiness and lethargy occur frequently in the elderly or in those with liver disorders. As with all barbiturates, the potential for tolerance, dependence and abuse is real when these drugs are taken regularly.

According to *AMA Drug Evaluations* (second edition, pg. 315), preparations containing a barbiturate and a bromoureide (e.g., carbromal) "have not been used as extensively as preparations containing only barbiturates. The bromoureides represent a class of weak sedatives that offer no advantage over similarly acting agents." It is clear that preparations such as Carbrital expose patients to an unnecessary drug agent (carbromal) and, therefore, unnecessary risks and unwanted extra expense. When taken regularly pentobarbital can lead to psychological and physical addiction.

---

*The amount of pentobarbital (an effective, short-acting sedative/hypnotic) included in Carbrital is sufficient to induce sleep or moderate sedation in most adults. To claim that alertness and sensory perception is not compromised by such medication strikes us as frankly deceptive.

- **Brand Name: CARBRITAL KAPSEALS HALF STRENGTH**
- **Manufacturer:** Parke-Davis
- **Use:** Anti-anxiety
- **Dosage Form:** Capsule
- **Administration:** Oral
- **Ingredients:** Pentobarbital sodium 49 mg, carbromal 130 mg (sedative/hypnotics).

CARBRITAL KAPSEALS HALF STRENGTH have components with exactly one-half the

dose strength of each component of Carbrital. The manufacturer stopped making this drug in late 1979, but it is still commercially available. When taken regularly, pentobarbital can lead to psychological and physical addiction.

See similar drug CARBRITAL KAPSEALS, pg. 68

- **Brand Name: CARDILATE**
- **Manufacturer:** Burroughs Wellcome
- **Use:** Heart pain (angina pectoris)
- **Dosage Form:** Tablet /Tablet /Tablet
- **Administration:** Oral / Sublingual / Chewable
- **Ingredients:** Erythrityl tetranitrate 5, 10 or 15 mg (coronary vasodilator).

CARDILATE is promoted and prescribed for the management and prevention of transient heart pain (angina pectoris) due to coronary artery disease. It is available in three distinct tablet forms: sublingual (dissolved under the tongue), chewable and oral (swallowed whole). According to the *AMA Drug Evaluations* (second edition, pg. 231), erythrityl tetranitrate, a vasodilating agent, is not useful for relief of an acute anginal attack when taken under the tongue. There is limited evidence that, as with nitroglycerin, it may be effective under the tongue as a preventive measure when taken just before situations known to precipitate anginal attacks, such as stress and physical exertion. However, most people who use this drug (and others like it) do so on a long-term basis. At present, there is insufficient evidence that the long-term oral administration of erythrityl tetranitrate will be of any real therapeutic value in managing or preventing angina.

Also see Part II: Drugs for Heart Pain

- **Brand Name: CARDILATE-P**
- **Manufacturer:** Burroughs Wellcome
- **Use:** Heart pain (angina pectoris)
- **Dosage Form:** Tablet
- **Administration:** Oral
- **Ingredients:** Erythrityl tetranitrate 10 mg (coronary vasodilator); phenobarbital 15 mg (sedative).

CARDILATE-P, as with Cardilate, not only lacks evidence of effectiveness, but also subjects the patient to the further danger of the addiction liability of a barbiturate (phenobarbital).

See similar drug CARDILATE, pg. 70

Also see Part II: Drugs for Heart Pain.

- **Brand Name: CARTRAX 10, 20**
- **Manufacturer:** Roerig
- **Use:** Heart pain (angina pectoris)
- **Dosage Form:** Tablet
- **Administration:** Oral
- **Ingredients:** Pentaerythritol tetranitrate 10 or 20 mg (coronary vasodilator); hydroxyzine hydrochloride 10 mg (antihistamine/tranquilizer).

CARTRAX, in both dosage strengths, is used to treat anginal pain (transient chest pain due to inadequate supply of blood and oxygen to the heart). Careful clinical studies fail to support the chronic use of pentaerythritol tetranitrate and similar nitrate vasodilators for the prevention of heart pain. Hydroxyzine, an antihistamine/tranquilizer included in Cartrax to provide an anti-anxiety effect, can cause drowsiness, loss of coordination, mental inattention and dizziness. The FDA presently considers Cartrax ineffective as a fixed-ratio combination.

Also see Part II: Drugs for Heart Pain

- **Brand Name: CENALENE**
- **Manufacturer:** Central
- **Use:** Central nervous system stimulation
- **Dosage Form:** Tablet /Elixir
- **Administration:** Oral/ Oral
- **Ingredients:** Pentylenetetrazol (stimulant/analeptic); thiamine hydrochloride, niacinamide, cyanocobalamin (vitamins); alcohol 15% (in elixir).

CENALENE is a multidrug combination comprised of a central nervous system stimulant and a number of vitamins (one with blood vessel dilating properties), and is used to enhance the mental and physical activity of elderly patients. It is also prescribed for vertigo and a disease of the inner ear (Meniere's). There is no evidence to support the drug's use for these conditions. Identical drugs include: Senoral-M.

See similar drug RU-VERT, pg. 172

- **Brand Name: CETACAINE**
- **Manufacturer:** Cetylite
- **Use:** Topical pain relief
- **Dosage Form:** Aerosol / Liquid / Ointment   Gel
- **Administration:** Spray / Topical / Topical   Topical
- **Ingredients:** Benzocaine 14%, butyl aminobenzoate 2%, tetracaine hydrochloride 2% (topical anesthetics); benzalkonium chloride 0.5% (antiseptic).

CETACAINE is a topical anesthetic used to numb mucous membranes (e.g., mouth and nose), and to control pain or gagging. The FDA has found it ineffective for its labeled indications.

- **Brand Name: CHARDONNA-2**
- **Manufacturer:** Rorer
- **Use:** Digestive disorders
- **Dosage Form:** Tablet
- **Administration:** Oral
- **Ingredients:** Belladonna extract 15 mg (antispasmodic/antisecretory); phenobarbital 15 mg (sedative).

CHARDONNA-2 is a fixed-combination product prescribed for a variety of gastrointestinal disorders, especially those with spasm. It is composed of a sedative (phenobarbital) and an antispasmodic/antisecretory component (belladonna extract). The question of whether combination drugs of this sort are useful in treating bowel disorders is highly controversial. There is no persuasive evidence that such fixed-combinations are in fact justified.

Sedatives, when administered on an individual basis, can alleviate a few symptoms, since some digestive problems can have an emotional basis. However, there is no reason to believe these combinations like Chardonna have any value in the treatment of ulcer. Chardonna suffers from all of the disadvantages of a fixed-combination. When taken regularly, phenobarbital can lead to psychological and physical addiction. Belladonna extract often causes blurring of vision, dryness of the mouth and throat, constipation and hesitancy of urination.

Also see Part II: Drugs for Digestive Disorders

- **Brand Name: CHLOROMYCETIN-HC**
- **Manufacturer:** Parke-Davis
- **Use:** Eye infection, inflammation
- **Dosage Form:** Solution
- **Administration:** Eye
- **Ingredients:** Chloramphenicol 1.25% (antibacterial); hydrocortisone 2.5% (corticosteroid).

CHLOROMYCETIN-HC is used to treat various eye infections, especially inflammatory conditions of the mucous membranes of the eye and lid that respond to the action of chloramphenicol, a broad-spectrum antibiotic. Hydrocortisone is included for the relief of inflammation associated with infection. The use of corticosteroids for the treatment of skin infections may be dangerous because they can either mask the evidence of infection or cause the spreading of infections.

WARNING: Chloramphenicol can cause serious and fatal blood disorders. Chloromycetin-HC should never be used and chloramphenicol alone should be limited to serious infections that do not respond to other antibacterial agents.

Also see Part II: Drugs Applied Directly to Skin, Eye or Ear

- **Brand Name: CHLORPHENIRAMINE MALEATE**
- **Manufacturer:** generic
- **Use:** Cold and allergy
- **Dosage Form:** Time-release tablet
- **Administration:** Oral
- **Ingredients:** Chlorpheniramine maleate 8 or 12 mg (antihistamine).

CHLORPHENIRAMINE MALEATE in the time-release form is promoted primarily for the treatment of hay fever and nasal congestion, as well as for other allergic conditions. At issue is whether the time-release form, not the actual drug itself, is effective. In general, chlorpheniramine is effective for treating allergies. The time-release form is not recommended because its action is unpredictable and its additional cost is unnecessary. Chlorpheniramine in all forms should not be used to treat the common cold, since there is no convincing evidence that antihistamines lessen cold symptoms. Chlorpheniramine can cause drowsiness, loss of coordination, mental inattention and dizziness.

Note: Chlorpheniramine maleate may now be purchased without a prescription. Identical drugs include: Allermine, Chlor-Hab, Chlorophen, Chlortab 8, Ciramine, Panahist, Phenetron.

Also see Part II: Drugs for Cough, Cold and Allergy

- **Brand Name: CHYMORAL**
- **Manufacturer:** Armour
- **Use:** Fluid retention
- **Dosage Form:** Enteric coated tablet
- **Administration:** Oral
- **Ingredients:** Trypsin, chymotrypsin (proteolytic enzymes).

CHYMORAL, as with a number of other oral enzyme products, is used primarily to control edema (fluid accumulation in tissues), inflammation (swelling, redness, heat and pain) associated with surgical or accidental trauma, infections and allergic manifestations. This product has not proven effective in these disorders. Identical drugs include: Chymoral-100.

- **Brand Name: CIRCUBID**
- **Manufacturer:** Merchant
- **Use:** Blood vessel disease (head and limbs)
- **Dosage Form:** Time-release capsule
- **Administration:** Oral
- **Ingredients:** Ethaverine hydrochloride 150 mg (vasodilator).

CIRCUBID is a time-release form of ethaverine hydrochloride. Circubid, like all ethaverine and papaverine based drug products, is prescribed primarily for treating disorders arising from insufficient blood flow to the head and limbs and, less frequently, for treating pain due to the lack of blood flow to the heart.

Ethaverine is a synthetic derivative of papaverine with the same actions, although ethaverine is roughly twice as potent. Thus Circubid is roughly equivalent in strength to Pavabid HP and Pavakey-300. Currently there is no evidence showing that any of these papaverine or ethaverine products are effective for their recommended uses and there is strong evidence that these drugs cause liver damage in many people. *(New Eng J Med* 281:1333-35 and 1364-65, 1969)

Also see Part II: Drugs for Circulatory Disorders of Head and Limbs

- Brand Name: **CLISTIN EXPECTORANT**
- **Manufacturer:** McNeil
- **Use:** Cough and cold
- **Dosage Form:** Syrup
- **Administration:** Oral
- **Ingredients:** Carbinoxamine maleate 2 mg (antihistamine); ammonium chloride 120 mg, potassium guaiacolsulfonate 60 mg, sodium citrate 120 mg (expectorants) per 5 ml; alcohol 0.3%.

CLISTIN EXPECTORANT is promoted for the symptomatic relief of cough in conditions such as the common cold, allergic asthma and acute bronchitis. However, there is no evidence that carbinoxamine, an antihistamine, is effective in suppressing the cough reflex. In fact, none of the ingredients has any cough-suppressing action. If an unproductive* cough is a problem, one should use an effective anti-cough agent such as dextromethorphan (more appropriate than codeine because it is non-narcotic). Clistin Expectorant is an expensive mixture that confers no therapeutic benefit. The FDA has rated Clistin Expectorant as ineffective for its labeled indications. Carbinoxamine can cause drowsiness, loss of coordination, mental inattention and dizziness; ammonium chloride can be harmful to patients with improperly functioning lungs, liver or kidneys.

*Coughs may actually be productive when one suffers from congested lungs and respiratory blockage, such as with pneumonia. When there is a lot of phlegm and mucus lodged in the breathing passages, the cough reflex is important and its suppression can be dangerous, especially for the older patient.

Also see Part II: Drugs for Cough, Cold and Allergy

- **Brand Name: CLISTIN R-A**
- **Manufacturer:** McNeil
- **Use:** Allergy
- **Dosage Form:** Time-release tablet
- **Administration:** Oral
- **Ingredients:** Carbinoxamine maleate 8 or 12 mg (antihistamine).

CLISTIN R-A is marketed for the treatment of hay fever and nasal congestion, as well as various other allergic conditions. The FDA has found Clistin R-A to be only "probably effective" for these indications. As with other "long-lasting" antihistamines, Clistin R-A is generally not recommended because its action may be uneven and the additional cost is unnecessary.

For the relief of various allergic conditions one would do best to purchase an antihistamine with fully effective ratings, such as diphenhydramine or chlorpheniramine in its generic form, instead of time-release. Carbinoxamine can cause drowsiness, loss of coordination, mental inattention and dizziness.

Also see Part II: Drugs for Cough, Cold and Allergy

- **Brand Name: COMBID SPANSULES**
- **Manufacturer:** Smith Kline & French
- **Use:** Digestive disorders
- **Dosage Forms:** Time-release capsule
- **Administration:** Oral
- **Ingredients:** Isopropamide iodide 5 mg (antispasmodic); prochlorperazine maleate 10 mg (tranquilizer).

COMBID SPANSULES are prescribed as supportive therapy in the treatment of peptic ulcer and "spastic colon." Even if the combination of ingredients found in Combid were acceptable, there is still the problem of its "time-release" form. This is unacceptable because the gut transit time is too unpredictable* to provide reliable drug availability for 12 hours. The time-release form also adds considerably to the cost of the drug.

There is no conclusive evidence that antispasmodic/antisecretory agents such as isopropamide iodide facilitate healing of ulcer or prevent complications; as a matter of fact, the *AMA Drug Evaluations* (first edition, pg. 594), cites Combid as an "irrational mixture." Combid includes the powerful anti-anxiety agent prochlorperazine. However, there is insufficient evidence that this component directly contributes to the intended action of Combid. Isopropamide often causes blurring of vision, dryness of the mouth and throat, constipation and hesitancy of urination. Identical drugs include: Com-Pro-Span Capsules, Prochlor-Iso Capsules.

*Such formulations often present the problem of uneven drug release—for instance, dumping all of the drug(s) into the blood stream rapidly, or releasing the ingredients too late to be effective. Responses are unacceptably variable with most time-release products.

Also see Part II: Drugs for Digestive Disorders

- **Brand Name: CO-PYRONIL**
- **Manufacturer:** Dista(Lilly)
- **Use:** Cold and allergy
- **Dosage Form:** Capsule / Suspension
- **Administration:** Oral /Oral
- **Ingredients:** Pyrrobutamine phosphate (antihistamine); cyclopentamine hydrochloride (sympathomimetic).

CO-PYRONIL is promoted for the symptomatic treatment of hay fever and nasal congestion, as well as a number of different allergic conditions. Co-Pyronil is composed of an antihistamine and cyclopentamine, a drug with adrenalin-like (sympathomimetic) effects. It is dubious that this combination is actually more efficacious than the individual components, or that both components are necessary; in common colds, the antihistamines have no proven effect. In general, antihistamines should not be purchased by their brand names, since the generic equivalents are considerably less expensive. Furthermore, as a general rule, one should avoid multicomponent cold and allergy remedies. Extra components are usually superfluous and add substantially to the cost. Cyclopentamine can cause or aggravate high blood pressure and commonly loses its effectiveness when used regularly while pyrrobutamine can cause drowsiness, loss of coordination, mental inattention and dizziness.

Also see Part II: Drugs for Cough, Cold and Allergy

- **Brand Name: CO-PYRONIL PEDIATRIC**
- **Manufacturer:** Dista(Lilly)
- **Use:** Cold and allergy
- **Dosage Form:** Capsule
- **Administration:** Oral
- **Ingredients:** Pyrrobutamine phosphate 7.5 mg (antihistamine); cyclopentamine hydrochloride 6.25 mg (sympathomimetic).

CO-PYRONIL PEDIATRIC is promoted for

the symptomatic treatment of hay fever and nasal congestion, as well as a number of other allergic conditions in children. Co-Pyronil Pediatric is composed of an antihistamine and cyclopentamine, a drug with adrenalin-like (sympathomimetic) effects. It is dubious that this combination is actually more efficacious than the individual components, or that both components are necessary; in common colds, the antihistamines have no proven effect. In general, antihistamines should not be purchased by their brand names, since the generic equivalents are considerably less expensive. Furthermore, as a general rule, one should avoid multi-component cold and allergy remedies. Extra components are usually superfluous and add substantially to the cost. Cyclopentamine can cause or aggravate high blood pressure and commonly loses its effectiveness when used regularly while pyrrobutamine can cause drowsiness, loss of coordination, mental inattention and dizziness.

Also see Part II: Drugs for Cough, Cold and Allergy

- **Brand Name: CORDRAN- N**
- **Manufacturer:** Dista(Lilly)
- **Use:** Skin disorders
- **Dosage Form:** Cream /Ointment
- **Administration:** Topical/ Topical
- **Ingredients:** Neomycin sulfate 0.5% (antibacterial); flurandrenolide 0.05%(corticosteroid).

CORDRAN-N is employed for the relief of the inflam-

matory manifestations of various skin disorders complicated by bacterial infections. The use of corticosteroids for the treatment of skin infections may be dangerous because they can either mask the evidence of infection or cause the spreading of infections. Neomycin commonly causes skin rashes and can sensitize people to other more important antibiotics.

See similar drug CALDECORT, pg. 67

Also see Part II: Drugs Applied Directly to Skin, Eye or Ear

- **Brand Name: COR-TAR-QUIN**
- **Manufacturer:** Dome
- **Use:** Skin disorders
- **Dosage Form:** Cream / Lotion
- **Administration:** Topical / Topical
- **Ingredients:** Hydrocortisone 0.25, 0.5 or 1% (corticosteroid); carbonis detergens (coal tar) 2%; diiodohydroxyquin 1% (anti-infective).

COR-TAR-QUIN is used primarily in the treatment of psoriasis, an inflammatory skin disease, and other skin disorders. This product contains coal tar, which can cause skin irritation and sensitivity to light.

Also see Part II: Drugs Applied Directly to Skin, Eye or Ear

- **Brand Name: CORTISPORIN CREAM**
- **Manufacturer:** Burroughs Wellcome
- **Use:** Skin infection, wound healing
- **Dosage Form:** Cream
- **Administration:** Topical
- **Ingredients:** Polymyxin B sulfate 10,000 u, neomycin sulfate .5%, gramacidin 0.25 mg (antibacterials); hydrocortisone acetate .5% (corticosteroid) per gram.

CORTISPORIN CREAM is promoted primarily to improve wound healing and resolution of skin infections. The use of corticosteroids for the treatment of skin infections may be dangerous because they can either mask the evidence of infection or cause the spreading of infections. Neomycin commonly causes skin rashes and can sensitize people to other more important antibiotics.

Also see Part II: Drugs Applied Directly to Skin, Eye or Ear

- **Brand Name: CORTISPORIN OINTMENT**
- **Manufacturer:** Burroughs Wellcome
- **Use:** Skin infection, wound healing
- **Dosage Form:** Ointment
- **Administration:** Topical
- **Ingredients:** Polymyxin B sulfate 5000 u, bacitracin 400 u, neomycin sulfate .5% (antibacterials); hydrocortisone 1% (corticosteroid) per gram.

CORTISPORIN OINTMENT, promoted

primarily to improve wound healing and prevent skin infections, is a mixture of three antibacterials and a steroid. The use of corticosteroids for the treatment of skin infections may be dangerous because they can either mask the evidence of infection or cause the spreading of infections. Neomycin commonly causes skin rashes and can sensitize people to other more important antibiotics.

Also see Part II: Drugs Applied Directly to Skin, Eye or Ear

- **Brand Name: CORTISPORIN OPHTHALMIC**
- **Manufacturer:** Burroughs Wellcome
- **Use:** Eye infection
- **Dosage Form:** Ointment / Suspension
- **Administration:** Eye / Eye
- **Ingredients:** Polymyxin B sulfate 5,000 or 10,000 u, neomycin sulfate 0.5%, bacitracin zinc 400 u [only in ointment] (antibacterials); hydrocortisone 1% (corticosteroid).

CORTISPORIN OPHTHALMIC is used

in the treatment of various eye and eyelid infections of bacterial and allergic origin. The use of corticosteroids for the treatment of eye infections may be dangerous because they either mask the evidence of infection or cause the spreading of infections. Neomycin commonly causes skin rashes and can sensitize people to other more important antibiotics. According to the *AMA Drug Evaluations* (first edition, pg. 526), Cortisporin Ophthalmic Ointment is an "irrational mixture" and combination products containing corticosteroids and antibiotics are "not recommended for the topical [external] treatment of ocular [eye] infections."

See similar drug NEO-CORTEF OPHTHALMIC, pg. 124

Also see Part II: Drugs Applied Directly to Skin, Eye or Ear

- Brand Name: **CYCLOSPASMOL**
- **Manufacturer:** Ives
- **Use:** Blood vessel disease (head and limbs)
- **Dosage Form:** Capsule/ Tablet
- **Administration:** Oral /Oral
- **Ingredients:** Cyclandelate 100, 200 or 400 mg (vasodilator).

CYCLOSPASMOL is promoted as adjunctive therapy for vascular disorders caused by decreased blood flow to the legs, arms and brain; inflammation of veins due to clots; leg cramps at night; and blanching of the fingers or hands in response to cold. Although this drug does relax the smooth muscle that lines medium-sized and small blood vessels in normal humans, there is no convincing evidence to support the manufacturer's claims that Cyclospasmol confers a therapeutic benefit to patients with peripheral vascular disease or cerebral (brain) vascular disease.

The *AMA Drug Evaluations* (third edition pg. 36) concludes that the efficacy of cyclandelate in these vascular disorders is "questionable." Identical drugs include: Cyclanfor, Cydel, Cyvaso, Cyvaso-400, Cyclandelate.

Also see Part II: Drugs for Circulatory Disorders of Head and Limbs

- Brand Name: **DAINITE**
- **Manufacturer:** Wallace
- **Use:** Asthma, respiratory disorders
- **Dosage Form:** Tablet
- **Administration:** Oral
- **Ingredients:** Aminophylline 200 mg, ephedrine hydrochloride 16 mg (bronchodilators); sodium pentobarbital 16 mg (sedative); benzocaine 16 mg (anesthetic); aluminum hydroxide 160 mg (antacid).

DAINITE is promoted and prescribed for the prevention and symptomatic treatment of asthma. One of the ingredients, benzocaine, a topical anesthetic, does nothing to relieve bronchial spasm or promote freer breathing. Aminophylline can be effective in the proper individualized dose, but the dose in Dainite may not be effective for many people. The only two ingredients in Dainite of any value in relieving the symptoms of asthma are aminophylline and ephedrine. However, ephedrine often loses its efficacy after continued use, and may cause or aggravate high blood pressure.

Pentobarbital, an effective sedative, has been added in an attempt to offset the common, unpleasant side effects of ephedrine, such as anxiety and rapid heartbeat. There is no evidence that it contributes to relieving the asthma symptoms or preventing them from occurring. Pentobarbital is a barbiturate, and its regular use can produce psychological and physical addiction.

- **Brand Name: DAINITE-KI**
- **Manufacturer:** Wallace
- **Use:** Asthma, respiratory disorders
- **Dosage Form:** Tablet
- **Administration:** Oral
- **Ingredients:** Aminophylline 200 mg, ephedrine hydrochloride 16 mg (bronchodilators); phenobarbital 16 mg (sedative); benzocaine 16 mg (anesthetic); aluminum hydroxide 160 mg (antacid); potassium iodide 325 mg (expectorant).

DAINITE-KI contains potassium iodide (KI), an agent that supposedly makes phlegm easier to cough up. However, there is no persuasive evidence that all of the ingredients in Dainite-KI add up to an effective asthma medicine.

Ephedrine can cause or aggravate high blood pressure and commonly loses its effectiveness when used regularly. There is no clinical evidence that phenobarbital is effective in the treatment of asthma. Aminophylline can be effective at the proper individualized dose, but the dose in this product may not be effective for many people. For the relief of most cases of asthma, aminophylline or another single-entity bronchodilating agent is preferred. When taken regularly, phenobarbital can lead to psychological and physical addiction.

See similar drug DAINITE, pg. 82

- **Brand Name: DARICON PB**
- **Manufacturer:** Beecham
- **Use:** Digestive disorders
- **Dosage Form:** Tablet
- **Administration:** Oral
- **Ingredients:** Oxyphencyclimine hydrochloride 5 mg (antispasmodic); phenobarbital 15 mg (sedative).

DARICON PB is used for a variety of digestive disorders but there is a dearth of evidence to support its clinical efficacy for these medical problems. There is no evidence that Daricon PB relieves ulcer pain or hastens healing. Most combination products of this type do not provide an adequate amount of either the antispasmodic/antisecretory drug or the sedative. Moreover, these components require greater individualization of dosage than most drugs, which further reduces the value of a fixed-combination of this type. When taken regularly phenobarbital can lead to psychological and physical addiction. Oxyphencyclimine often causes blurring of vision, dryness of the mouth and throat, constipation and hesitancy of urination.

Also see Part II: Drugs for Digestive Disorders

- **Brand Name: DEANER**
- **Manufacturer:** Riker
- **Use:** Anti-depressant, learning problems, behavioral problems
- **Dosage Form:** Tablet
- **Administration:** Oral
- **Ingredients:** Deanol acetamidobenzoate 25 or 100 mg (psychostimulant).

DEANER is promoted and prescribed for patients (often children) with learning problems (including short attention span) and behavioral problems (hyperkinesis, a condition characterized by distractability and constant physical activity). Deaner is also employed as an anti-depressant for patients suffering from neurotic disorders and chronic fatigue. However, this drug is presently considered "lacking in substantial evidence of effectiveness." According to the *AMA Drug Evaluations* (second edition, pg. 30), the effectiveness of deanol acetamidobenzoate as an "antidepressant or in the management of children with behavioral and learning problems has not been demonstrated conclusively."

Drug therapy for the so-called "hyperactive child" syndrome is a controversial issue and is probably inappropriate in many cases even if an "effective" drug is used.

- **Brand Name: DECA-DURABOLIN**
- **Manufacturer:** Organon
- **Use:** Bone, growth disorders
- **Dosage Form:** Solution
- **Administration:** Injection
- **Ingredients:** Nandrolone decanoate 50 or 100 mg (androgenic steroid).

DECA-DURABOLIN is a weak androgen (male hormone) used primarily as adjunctive therapy in the treatment of senile and post-menopausal bone disorders (progressive loss of bone mass) and various arthritic conditions. It has been used in the management of certain growth disorders in children but therapy can result in irreversible adverse effects. The National Academy of Sciences-National Research Council cautions that the use of this type of hormone (androgenic steroid) in the treatment of progressive bone disease is without proven value as a primary therapy.

Although this use is not to be found in the drug's approved package labeling, some 15 percent of the Deca-Durabolin prescriptions are given to patients with serious arthritic conditions, such as rheumatoid arthritis, for which the drug has no proven benefit. Its side effects can include masculinization of females. Identical drugs include: Anabolin LA 100, Androlone-D 50, Androlone-D 100, Nandrolate.

See similar drug WINSTROL, pg. 188

- **Brand Name: DECASPRAY**
- **Manufacturer:** Merck Sharp & Dohme
- **Use:** Skin disorders
- **Dosage Form:** Aerosol
- **Administration:** Topical
- **Ingredients:** Dexamethasone (corticosteroid); isopropyl myristate.

DECASPRAY is used in the treatment of certain skin diseases. One of the two active ingredients in this combination, dexamethasone, is employed chiefly to eliminate or control the inflammatory or allergic effects of these dermatological, or skin, disorders. Because dexamethasone is fluorinated, skin eruptions can occur with protracted use. Identical drugs include: Aeroseb-Dex.

Also see Part II: Drugs Applied Directly to Skin, Eye or Ear

- **Brand Name: DECLOSTATIN**
- **Manufacturer:** Lederle
- **Use:** Bacterial and fungal infection
- **Dosage Form:** Capsule
- **Administration:** Oral
- **Ingredients:** Demeclocycline hydrochloride 150 mg (antibacterial); nystatin 250,000 u (antifungal).

DECLOSTATIN is a fixed-combination product used to treat infections of bacterial and fungal origin. Demeclocycline is a broad-spectrum antibiotic related to tetracycline. It can sensitize patients to sunlight and sometimes can cause severe blistering. Moreover, it is preferable to give the antifungal agent, nystatin, separately if needed for fungal infection. Nystatin can cause nausea and vomiting.

The rationale behind the use of fixed-ratio combinations such as Declostatin is faulty. The nystatin element is added to prevent the onset of a "superinfection" by yeast and other fungi of the intestinal tract which might occur following the use of a broad-spectrum antibiotic. The idea is that when an antibiotic kills most intestinal bacteria, the antibiotic-resistant yeasts have a much better opportunity to grow. However, this type of superinfection rarely occurs. Furthermore, the amount of nystatin used in fixed-combinations such as Declostatin is insufficient to prevent such an occurrence. If a superinfection of yeast does set in, it is best to treat it *separately* with appropriate drugs.

See similar drug MYSTECLIN F, pg. 122

- **Brand Name: DECLOSTATIN-300**
- **Manufacturer:** Lederle
- **Use:** Bacterial and fungal infection
- **Dosage Form:** Tablet
- **Administration:** Oral
- **Ingredients:** Demeclocycline hydrochloride 300 mg (antibacterial); nystatin 500,000 u (antifungal).

DECLOSTATIN-300 is a fixed-combination used to eliminate infections of bacterial and fungal origin. It is also widely prescribed to prevent the overgrowth of intestinal fungi during broad-spectrum antibacterial treatment with demeclocycline, a derivative of common tetracycline.

Declostatin-300, like most fixed-combination regimens of its kind, contains nystatin in minimal dosage. Moreover, the administration of such mixtures for preventive purposes is poor medical practice. Both ingredients should be given separately if actually required, with dosages adjusted to the individual patient's needs. Demeclocycline can sensitize the skin to sunlight and cause severe blistering. Nystatin can cause nausea and vomiting.

See similar drug DECLOSTATIN, pg. 85 and MYSTECLIN F, pg. 122

- **Brand Name: DEPROL**
- **Manufacturer:** Wallace
- **Use:** Depression therapy
- **Dosage Form:** Tablet
- **Administration:** Oral
- **Ingredients:** Meprobamate 400 mg (tranquilizer); benactyzine hydrochloride 1 mg (antidepressant).

DEPROL has been classified by the FDA as "lacking substantial evidence of effectiveness" in the management of depression, both acute (reactive) and chronic. It is used in depressions that are accompanied by anxiety, insomnia, agitation or upset stomach. This drug is a fixed-combination, comprised of the antidepressant benactyzine hydrochloride and the tranquilizer meprobamate. The *AMA Drug Evaluations* (second edition, pg.323) states that such mixtures have a questionable rationale. When two or more agents with similar indications are combined, the patient is exposed to the possible development of increased adverse drug reactions, often without any compensating advantage.

Deprol fails to meet the federal standards for effectiveness. Better, effective medicines are available for depression when medicines are needed. (Antidepressant drugs should always be taken in conjunction with psychotherapeutic counseling, and should never be considered the primary therapy.)

WARNING: The use of minor tranquilizers such as meprobamate (Miltown), chlordiazepoxide (Librium), diazepam (Valium) or similar drugs during pregnancy should be avoided because of increased risk of damage to the developing fetus. One must consider the possibility of pregnancy when beginning minor tranquilizer therapy. In the case of combination drugs such as Deprol, use at any time is unwarranted.

- **Brand Name: DEXAMYL**
- **Manufacturer:** Smith Kline & French
- **Use:** Treatment of obesity
- **Dosage Form:** Elixir   Tablet / Spansule
- **Administration:** Oral   Oral /Oral
- **Ingredients:** Amobarbital (sedative/barbiturate); dextroamphetamine (stimulant).

DEXAMYL, a fixed-ratio mixture of an amphetamine and a sedative, is currently considered by the FDA as lacking in substantial evidence of effectiveness for the treatment of overweight patients.

Amobarbital, included in Dexamyl to offset stimulation from the amphetamine, contributes no significant benefit. Though it is present in a small quantity, this barbiturate may at times cause sedation (sleepiness), and it can cause serious drug addiction as well.

Amphetamines, long used as appetite suppressants, are also known as "speed" and have profound side effects, such as high blood pressure, anxiety and trouble in sleeping. They carry significant risks and are considered marginally effective, at best, only for very short-term weight control (12 weeks). There is no good evidence that patients keep the weight off following the drug therapy. According to the FDA Advisory Committee studying amphetamines: "The natural history of obesity is measured in years, whereas the studies cited are restricted to a few weeks' duration; thus, the total impact of drug-induced weight loss over that of diet must be considered *clinically trivial.* The limited usefulness of these agents must be measured against any possible risk factor inherent in their use" (emphasis added). Recently, however, the FDA announced its decision that single-entity amphetamines should no longer be labeled as approved for the treatment of obesity, and began efforts to implement that proposal. This decision was prompted by much evidence of continuing misuse and abuse of amphetamines and severe risks of dependence. These harmful effects create an unfavorable benefit-to-risk ratio when compared to the trivial effect the drugs have on reducing weight.

In addition to cosmetic and social motivations, doctors often urge overweight patients to reduce because of the increased risk of developing heart disease and diabetes associated with obesity. Yet, one of the principal risks associated with amphetamine use is the increased stress on the heart.

Dexamyl is clearly an "irrational" mixture and should have been removed from the market long ago. Combining an "upper" and a "downer" is dangerous and entirely unwarranted. The FDA has ruled that such mixtures are inappropriate and has acted to remove them from the market; yet some, like Dexamyl and Eskatrol, remain available.

Although the manufacturers stopped producing Dexamyl as of early 1980, the drug is still available through commercial channels.

WARNING: The chronic use of amphetamines may lead to drug dependence and abuse. Their potential for abuse is related to their action as a central nervous system stimulant. They can produce intense psychological dependence and severe social dysfunction.

- **Brand Name: DIANABOL**
- **Manufacturer:** Ciba
- **Use:** Bone, growth disorders
- **Dosage Form:** Tablet
- **Administration:** Oral
- **Ingredients:** Methandrostenolone 2.5 or 5 mg (androgenic steroid).

DIANABOL, a weak male hormone, is used as adjunctive therapy in the treatment of senile and post-menopausal bone diseases (progressive decrease in total bone mass). It is also sometimes used in the management of certain growth disorders in children, but it can cause masculinization in girls or women. The FDA stresses that Dianabol is without value as a primary therapy for progressive bone disorder (osteoporosis) and that equal or greater consideration should be given to diet, calcium balance, physical therapy and other good health-promoting measures. Like all steroids, a significant portion of the prescriptions written each year are for conditions not included as part of the FDA approved drug labeling. Approximately 15 percent of the annual prescriptions for Dianabol are given for patients with various serious arthritic conditions, although this use is inappropriate. Using these anabolic steroids to stimulate appetite is also improper, although some doctors still do so.

See similar drug WINSTROL, pg. 188

- **Brand Name: DIMETANE EXPECTORANT**
- **Manufacturer:** Robins
- **Use:** Cough, cold, allergy
- **Dosage Form:** Syrup
- **Administration:** Oral
- **Ingredients:** Brompheniramine maleate 2 mg (antihistamine); phenylephrine hydrochloride 5 mg, phenylpropanolamine hydrochloride 5 mg (sympathomimetics); guaifenesin 100 mg (expectorant) per 5 ml; alcohol 3.5%.

DIMETANE EXPECTORANT, which is prescribed for cough due to common cold and other respiratory disorders, has been found by FDA to lack substantial evidence of effectiveness as a fixed-combination. As with most fixed-dosage combination products, there are numerous disadvantages in using it. Not all ingredients are present in optimal therapeutic amounts; nor do all have appropriate therapeutic effects. As a general rule, multidrug "shotgun" preparations should be avoided. Phenylephrine and phenylpropanolamine can cause or aggravate high blood pressure and commonly lose their effectiveness when used regularly while brompheniramine can cause drowsiness, loss of coordination, mental inattention and dizziness. Identical drugs include: Midatane Expectorant, Normatane Expectorant, Puretane Expectorant, Spentane Expectorant.

Also see Part II: Drugs for Cough, Cold and Allergy

- **Brand Name: DIMETANE EXPECTORANT-DC**
- **Manufacturer:** Robins
- **Use:** Cough, cold, allergy
- **Dosage Form:** Syrup
- **Administration:** Oral
- **Ingredients:** Brompheniramine maleate 2 mg (antihistamine); phenylephrine hydrochloride 5 mg, phenylpropanolamine hydrochloride 5 mg (sympathomimetics); guaifenesin 100 mg (expectorant); codeine phosphate 10 mg (antitussive).

DIMETANE EXPECTORANT-DC is another expensive example of the "shotgun" approach to the treatment of cough. While the DC product contains an effective anti-cough agent, codeine phosphate, there is no substantial evidence to demonstrate this drug's clinical efficacy as a fixed-combination. For the relief of cough, one should use generic dextromethorphan, a non-narcotic cough suppressant, if anything. Phenylephrine and phenyl-propanolamine can cause or aggravate high blood pressure and commonly lose their effectiveness when used regularly while brom-pheniramine can cause drowsiness, loss of coordination, mental inattention and dizziness. Codeine often causes drowsiness and constipation and is psychologically and physically addicting when taken regularly. Identical drugs include: Midatane DC Expectorant, Normatane DC Expectorant w/Codeine, Puretane Expectorant DC, Spentane DC Expectorant.

See similar drug DIMETANE EXPECTORANT, pg. 89

Also see Part II: Drugs for Cough, Cold and Allergy

- Brand Name: **DIMETAPP ELIXIR**
- **Manufacturer:** Robins
- **Use:** Cold and allergy
- **Dosage Form:** Elixir
- **Administration:** Oral
- **Ingredients:** Brompheniramine maleate 4 mg (antihistamine); phenylephrine hydrochloride 5 mg, phenylpropanolamine hydro-chloride 5 mg (sympathomimetics) per 5 ml; alcohol 2.3%.

DIMETAPP ELIXIR is promoted for the sympto-matic relief of hay fever and other perennial allergic nasal inflamma-tions. It is also sold and used as a fixed-combination in the relief of upper respiratory infection, nasal congestion, ear infection, bron-chitis and sore throat. However, for these disorders there is no sub-stantial evidence of Dimetapp's efficacy. Phenylephrine and phenyl-propanolamine can cause or aggravate high blood pressure and commonly lose their effectiveness when used regularly while brom-pheniramine can cause drowsiness, loss of coordination, mental inat-tention and dizziness. Identical drugs include: Bromalix Elixir, Bromepaph Elixir, Brompheniramine Compound Elixir, Brotapp Elixir, Eldatapp Liquid, Histatapp Elixir, Midatap Elixir, Norma-tane Elixir, Puretapp Elixir, Spentapp Elixir, Tagatap Syrup, Taltapp Elixir, Veltap Elixir, Westapp Elixir.

Also see Part II: Drugs for Cough, Cold and Allergy

- **Brand Name: DIMETAPP EXTENTABS**
- **Manufacturer:** Robins
- **Use:** Cold, allergy, respiratory disorders
- **Dosage Form:** Time-release tablet
- **Administration:** Oral
- **Ingredients:** Brompheniramine maleate 12 mg (antihistamine); phenylephrine hydrochloride 15 mg, phenylpropanolamine hydrochloride 15 mg (sympathomimetics).

DIMETAPP EXTENTABS have been classified by the FDA as lacking substantial evidence of effectiveness as a fixed-combination for the symptomatic relief of allergic manifestations of various upper respiratory illnesses.

The time-release form is of dubious efficacy; its use is not recommended because of uneven action and unnecessary additional cost. Phenylephrine and phenylpropanolamine can cause or aggravate high blood pressure and commonly lose their effectiveness when used regularly while brompheniramine can cause drowsiness, loss of coordination, mental inattention and dizziness. Identical drugs include: Bromepaph Tablets, Bromophen Tablets, Bromatapp Tablets, Eldatapp Tablets, Histatapp Tablets, Midatap Tablets, Normatane Tablets, Puretapp Tablets, Spentapp Tablets, Tagatap Tablets, Taltapp Duradisks.

See similar drug: DIMETAPP ELIXIR, pg. 90
Also see Part II: Drugs for Cough, Cold and Allergy

- **Brand Name: DISOPHROL**
- **Manufacturer:** Schering
- **Use:** Cold and allergy
- **Dosage Form:** Time-release tablet / Tablet
- **Administration:** Oral / Oral
- **Ingredients:** Dexbrompheniramine maleate 2 or 6 mg (antihistamine); pseudoephedrine sulfate 60 or 120 mg (sympathomimetic).

DISOPHROL is marketed principally for the symptomatic treatment of seasonal and perennial allergic nasal inflammation and nasal congestion. This is a poor choice of drugs for the relief of these symptoms.

In general, the use of fixed-combination products is poor medical practice. Disophrol is expensive, and can easily be replaced for treatment of allergy with a generic antihistamine like diphenhydramine (Benadryl) or chlorpheniramine (Chlor-Trimeton). For the relief of nasal congestion, phenylephrine (Neo-Synephrine) nose drops are preferable if a stuffy nose is very bothersome. Pseudoephedrine can cause or aggravate high blood pressure and commonly loses its effectiveness when used regularly, while dexbrompheniramine can cause drowsiness, loss of coordination, mental inattention and dizziness. Identical drugs include: Drixoral.

Also see Part II: Drugs for Cough, Cold and Allergy

- **Brand Name: DIUTENSEN**
- **Manufacturer:** Wallace
- **Use:** High blood pressure
- **Dosage Form:** Tablet
- **Administration:** Oral
- **Ingredients:** Methyclothiazide 2.5 mg (diuretic); cryptenamine tannate 2 mg (antihypertensive).

DIUTENSEN has been rated by the FDA as an ineffective fixed-combination for use in basic high blood pressure (hypertensive) therapy and for essential hypertension of all grades of severity. As a rule, fixed-combination products should not be used for the treatment of hypertension, because this disease requires therapy designed to meet the needs of individual patients.

Cryptenamine tannate, a drug of highly questionable effectiveness in the treatment of high blood pressure, must be adjusted carefully because of the narrow margin between therapeutic and toxic doses. Because of this, the *AMA Drug Evaluations* (first edition, pg. 40) regards Diutensen as an "irrational" combination, and the NAS-NRC saw fit to classify it as ineffective.

WARNING: This fixed-combination drug is not indicated for initial therapy of hypertension.

- **Brand Name: DONNATAL**
- **Manufacturer:** Robins
- **Use:** Digestive disorders
- **Dosage Forms:** Tablet / Capsule / Elixir
- **Administration:** Oral / Oral / Oral
- **Ingredients:** Hyoscyamine sulfate, atropine sulfate, hyoscine hydrobromide (antispasmodic/antisecretories); phenobarbital (sedative).

DONNATAL in its various forms is promoted as back-up therapy for patients with stomach ulcer, irritable bowel syndrome or other gastrointestinal problems. However, there is a lack of adequate evidence of efficacy for all forms of Donnatal.

According to *AMA Drug Evaluations* (first edition, pg. 594), this is an "irrational mixture." *The New Handbook of Prescription Drugs* states that "for most adults the hyoscyamine and hyoscine components can be little more than placebos in these small amounts and the dosage of atropine sulfate is also very small."[1] There is also no clinical evidence that antispasmodic/antisecretory drugs, most of Donnatal's ingredients, promote the healing of stomach ulcer, decrease recurrences or prevent complications. The *Handbook* states "[i]f there is any instance of widespread, thoughtless prescription practice, it is with Donnatal."[2] This seems to be a fair indictment of virtually all of the similar antispasmodic/antisecretory sedative combinations found in this guide. When taken regularly, the sedative phenobarbital can lead to psychological and physical addiction. Hyoscyamine, atropine and hyoscine often cause blurring of vision, dryness of the mouth and throat, constipation and hesitancy of urination. Identical drugs include: Antispasmodic Elixir, Donna-Phenal Elixir, Donna-Sed Elixir, Genespas-PB Elixir, Hyosophen Capsules, Hyosophen Tablets, Sedralex Elixir, Sedralex Tablets, Setamine Liquid, Setamine Tablets, Spalix Elixir, Spalix Tablets, Spasmolin Capsules, Spasmolin Tablets, Spasmophen Elixir.

[1] Burack R, Fox FJ. *The New Handbook of Prescription Drugs,* revised edition, Ballantine, 194: 1975.
[2] Ibid, 195.

Also see Part II: Drugs for Digestive Disorders

- **Brand Name: DONNATAL EXTENTABS**
- **Manufacturer:** Robins
- **Use:** Digestive disorders
- **Dosage Form:** Time-release tablets
- **Administration:** Oral
- **Ingredients:** Hyoscyamine sulfate 0.31 mg, atropine sulfate 0.058 mg, hyoscine hydrobromide 0.0195 mg (antispasmodic/antisecretories); phenobarbital 48.6 mg (sedative).

DONNATAL EXTENTABS are prescribed

for the same gastrointestinal conditions as is Donnatal. Extentabs are even more costly than regular Donnatal. In general, time-release pills such as Donnatal Extentabs are not recommended, as their "longer-action" is uneven.

Although some patients may benefit from the use of a sedative to help alleviate the anxiety that may in part be responsible for aggravating intestinal and stomach problems, this should be decided on an individual basis. A sedative, if used at all, should be administered separately at a dose adjusted to the patient's specific needs. The amount of phenobarbital (48.6 mg) included in Donnatal Extentabs is a large dose, and will likely cause pronounced drowsiness. Donnatal Extentabs are another prime example of the dangers and drawbacks of rigid, fixed-ratio combination drugs. If taken regularly, phenobarbital can lead to psychological and physical addiction. Hyoscyamine, atropine and hyoscine often cause blurring of vision, dryness of the mouth and throat, constipation and hesitancy of urination. Identical drugs include: Hyosophen T.D. Capsules.

Also see Part II: Drugs for Digestive Disorders

- **Brand Name: DONPHEN**
- **Manufacturer:** Lemmon
- **Use:** Digestive disorders
- **Dosage Form:** Tablet / Capsule
- **Administration:** Oral / Oral
- **Ingredients:** Hyoscyamine sulfate 0.1 mg, atropine sulfate 0.02 mg, hyoscine hydrobromide 0.006 mg (antispasmodic/antisecretories); phenobarbital 15 mg (sedative).

DONPHEN is recommended by the manufacturer to treat digestive disorders, kidney pain, nausea and vomiting connected with pregnancy, menstrual pain, motion sickness, insomnia and other conditions. It is one of a large group of fixed-combinations (antispasmodic/antisecretory and sedative) products used for a variety of problems primarily those involving the digestive system. There is no compelling justification for using this product for nausea, motion sickness or insomnia since none of the individual components are drugs of choice, and single-entity drugs are preferred. There is no satisfactory evidence that Donphen and related products have any therapeutic value in the healing of stomach ulcer or in treating intestinal disease. When taken regularly phenobarbital can lead to psychological and physical addiction. Hyoscyamine, atropine and hyoscine often cause blurring of vision, dryness of the mouth and throat, constipation and hesitancy of urination.

See similar drug DONNATAL, pg. 93

Also see Part II: Drugs for Digestive Disorders

- **Brand Name: DUOTRATE PLATEAU CAPS**
- **Manufacturer:** Marion
- **Use:** Heart pain (angina pectoris)
- **Dosage Form:** Time-release capsule
- **Administration:** Oral
- **Ingredients:** Pentaerythritol tetranitrate 30 or 45 mg (coronary vasodilator).

DUOTRATE is sold and used for the management, prevention and/or treatment of transient heart pain due to inadequate blood supply to the heart muscle (angina). There is no convincing clinical evidence of the efficacy of this product as long-term oral therapy for angina pectoris. At present, no careful clinical studies justify the regular use of pentaerythritol tetranitrate or similar oral nitrate vasodilators in preventing angina. Identical drugs include: Antora T.D., Desatrate 30, Kaytrate-30, Neo-Corovas-30 Tymcaps, Pentraspan-30, P.E.T.N., Rate-T-30.

Also see Part II: Drugs for Heart Pain

- **Brand Name: D-VASO**
- **Manufacturer:** Dunhall
- **Use:** Central nervous system stimulation
- **Dosage Form:** Capsule / Syrup
- **Administration:** Oral /Oral
- **Ingredients:** Pentylenetetrazol (stimulant/analeptic); niacin (vitamin/vasodilator); dimenhydrinate (antihistamine); alcohol 18% (in syrup).

D-VASO is an irrational, ineffective combination administered in the attempt to enhance the mental and physical activity of elderly patients and to relieve the dizziness that often accompanies old age. The principal ingredient, pentylenetetrazol, is a brain stimulant that has been used in the past, with minimal success, to stimulate breathing. However, there is no evidence to substantiate the efficacy of pentylenetetrazol, whether alone or in combination products such as D-Vaso, for the treatment of senility, mental depression, vertigo or a disease of the inner ear (Meniere's). The antihistamine dimenhydrinate has no proven benefit in the normal lightheadedness sometimes associated with old age, and may cause drowsiness, loss of coordination, mental inattention and dizziness. According to the *AMA Drug Evaluations* (second edition, pg. 379), the use of pentylenetetrazol-containing drugs has no place in modern medicine. Identical drugs include: Verticon.

See similar drug RU-VERT, pg. 172

- Brand Name: **ENARAX 5, 10**
- **Manufacturer:** Beecham
- **Use:** Digestive disorders
- **Dosage Form:** Tablet
- **Administration:** Oral
- **Ingredients:** Oxyphencyclimine hydrochloride 5 or 10 mg (antispasmodic/antisecretory); hydroxyzine hydrochloride 25 mg (sedative).

ENARAX is sold and prescribed for a variety of digestive disorders, including stomach ulcers. The antispasmodic/antisecretory agent oxyphencyclimine in this preparation acts to decrease the rate of acid secretion in the stomach and slows down the movement of food through the intestinal tract. Both of these effects are thought to relieve some of the pain of stomach ulcer and other digestive disorders. But at this point there is no conclusive evidence that antispasmodic/antisecretory drugs facilitate the healing of ulcers or prevent complications or recurrences. Even their effect in slowing intestinal overactivity is minimal. Enarax contains an additional ingredient, hydroxyzine, a potent sedative that fails to confer significant benefit to the patient. At present, there is no convincing evidence that such combinations are rational therapy for digestive disorders. Oxyphencyclimine often causes blurring of vision, dryness of the mouth and throat, constipation and hesitancy of urination. Identical drugs include: Vistrax 5, 10.

Also see Part II: Drugs for Digestive Disorders

- **Brand Name: EQUAGESIC**
- **Manufacturer:** Wyeth
- **Use:** Pain relief and anxiety
- **Dosage Form:** Tablet
- **Administration:** Oral
- **Ingredients:** Meprobamate 150 mg (tranquilizer); ethoheptazine citrate 75 mg (analgesic); acetylsalicylic acid 250 mg (analgesic/antipyretic).

EQUAGESIC is used primarily for the treatment of pain accompanied by tension and/or anxiety in patients with musculo-skeletal disease or tension headache.

In the treatment of muscle pain, a hot bath and 2 aspirin tablets will be at least as effective an analgesic (pain reliever) as Equagesic. According to the *AMA Drug Evaluations* (first edition, pg. 186), Equagesic is an "irrational mixture," the "analgesic effect of ethoheptazine is questionable, and there is no conclusive evidence that meprobamate enhances analgesic effectiveness of aspirin alone." Identical drugs include: Meprogesic.

WARNING: The use of minor tranquilizers such as meproba-mate (Miltown), chlordiazepoxide (Librium), diazepam (Valium) or similar drugs during pregnancy should be avoided because of increased risk of damage to the developing fetus. One must consider the possibility of pregnancy when beginning minor tranquilizer therapy. In the case of combination drugs such as Equagesic, use at any time is unwarranted.

- **Brand Name: ESGIC**
- **Manufacturer:** Gilbert
- **Use:** Pain relief
- **Dosage Form:** Tablet
- **Administration:** Oral
- **Ingredients:** Isobutylallylbarbituric acid 50 mg (sedative); acetaminophen 325 mg (analgesic); caffeine 40 mg (stimulant).

ESGIC is recommended by the manufacturer for pain, nervous tension, and sleeplessness associated with pain, headache, or general malaise. It is also prescribed for reduction of fever. Of the three ingredients in Esgic, acetaminophen is the only substance with analgesic properties of proven effectiveness. The sedative isobutylallylbarbituric acid allegedly enhances the analgesic efficacy of the product, but the evidence is unconvincing.

Very few properly controlled studies have been conducted to define what patients, if any, might benefit from combinations like Esgic, or to prove that such mixtures do, in fact, provide greater symptomatic benefit than an analgesic alone (either aspirin or acetaminophen). If a sedative is considered absolutely necessary, it should be given separately rather than in a fixed-combination. For mild to moderate pain, aspirin or acetaminophen alone is preferred. When taken regularly isobutylallylbarbituric acid can lead to psychological and physical addiction.

See similar drug SYNALGOS, pg. 174

- **Brand Name: ESKATROL SPANSULES**
- **Manufacturer:** Smith Kline & French
- **Use:** Treatment of obesity
- **Dosage Form:** Time-release capsule
- **Administration:** Oral
- **Ingredients:** Prochlorperazine maleate 7.5 mg (sedative/tranquilizer); dextroamphetamine sulfate 15 mg (stimulant).

ESKATROL SPANSULES are used in weight control therapy. This appetite-suppressing drug is a combination of a stimulant (amphetamine) and a sedative. Eskatrol is presently considered lacking in substantial evidence of effectiveness. Moreover, it has the well-recognized disadvantage of combination drugs in that adjustment of the doses of component drugs is impossible.

Dextroamphetamine is also known as "speed." While this class of drugs (amphetamines) has been used to control weight, they are widely abused for their stimulant effects. The effectiveness of amphetamines for control of obesity beyond the very short-term (12 weeks) is highly questionable. These drugs carry considerable risks, while offering no long-term benefit.

Dextroamphetamine is classified as a Schedule II drug under the Controlled Substances Act, meaning no refills are allowed. A major tranquilizer, in this case prochlorperazine, has been added to the amphetamine, supposedly to provide relief from emotional stress felt by the overweight patient attempting to lose weight. This combination is not only ineffective, but also dangerous. Although the tranquilizer is present in a sufficiently small dose to avoid a predominating sedative action, this is always a possibility. To use a combination of an "upper" and a "downer," both of which carry significant risks, is asking for trouble. Fixed-ratio combinations like Eskatrol have all been rated less-than-effective by the National Academy of Sciences-National Research Council (NAS-NRC) and should have been removed from the market long ago.

Adverse reactions may include psychological and, rarely, physical dependence in susceptible individuals, as well as insomnia, restlessness, nervousness, and dizziness. Psychosis (insanity) may occur with large doses. Cardiovascular symptoms may include increased pulse rate, high blood pressure, headache and chest pain.

Recently, the FDA concluded that *single-entity* amphetamines should no longer be labeled as approved for the treatment of obesity, and began efforts to implement that decision. The decision was prompted by plentiful evidence that the continuing misuse and abuse of amphetamines, the severe risk of dependence and the harmful effects that they present, create an unfavorable benefit-to-risk ratio when compared to the trivial effect they have on reducing weight.

WARNING: The chronic use of amphetamines may lead to drug dependence and abuse. Their potential for abuse is related to their action as a central nervous system stimulant. They can produce intense psychological dependence and severe social dysfunction.

- **Brand Name: ETHATAB**
- **Manufacturer:** Meyer
- **Use:** Blood vessel disease (head and limbs)
- **Dosage Form:** Tablet
- **Administration:** Oral
- **Ingredients:** Ethaverine hydrochloride 100 mg (vasodilator).

ETHATAB is promoted and prescribed for the treatment of a variety of disorders associated with insufficient blood flow. These include conditions involving the brain (arteriosclerosis), the extremities (cramping and leg pain) and the coronary arteries (angina pectoris). Ethaverine is a synthetic derivative of papaverine that has virtually the same drug action, although ethaverine is roughly twice as potent. However, there is no convincing evidence that the oral forms of ethaverine and papaverine have any therapeutic value for

100

the above conditions. Futhermore, there is strong evidence that these drugs can cause liver damage in many people. *(New Eng J Med 281:1333-35 and 1364-65, 1969)*. Identical drugs include: Ethaquin, Ethav, Laverin.

Also see Part II: Drugs for Circulatory Disorders of Head and Limbs

- **Brand Name: F-E-P CREAME**
- **Manufacturer:** Boots
- **Use:** Skin disorders
- **Dosage Form:** Cream
- **Administration:** Topical
- **Ingredients:** Iodochlorhydroxyquin 3% (anti-infective); hydrocortisone 1% (corticosteroid); pramoxine hydrochloride 0.5% (anesthetic).

F-E-P CREAME is used to treat a wide variety of skin disorders involving inflammation, fungal (yeast) infection and/or bacterial infection. For treatment of fungal infection one should use an antifungal agent such as nystatin or amphotericin B. Iodochlorhydroxyquin may be called for in the case of certain localized fungal infections that are complicated by bacterial infections since the drug has both antibacterial and antifungal activities (*AMA Drug Evaluations* second edition, pg. 602). In these cases the generic single-entity drug should be used. The use of corticosteroids for the treatment of skin infections may be dangerous because they can either mask the evidence of infection or cause the spreading of infections.

If hydrocortisone is needed for non-infectious skin conditions, such as inflammation, it should be administered by itself under close medical supervision. Identical drugs include: Dermarex, G.M.D., Iodosone, Quinsone, Stera-Form , Vio-Hydrosone.

Also see Part II: Drugs Applied Directly to Skin, Eye or Ear

- **Brand Name: FOLBESYN**
- **Manufacturer:** Lederle
- **Use:** Vitamin deficiency
- **Dosage Form:** Solution
- **Administration:** Injection
- **Ingredients:** Vitamins B-1, B-2, niacinamide, pantothenate, B-6, C, B-12, folic acid (vitamins).

FOLBESYN is used in preventing or treating vitamin deficiencies in certain disease states or post-operative conditions. As currently formulated, this parenteral (injectable) multi-vitamin preparation has been deemed ineffective by the FDA. The FDA asserts that there *is* a medical need for these all-inclusive vitamin products for various clinical conditions and that the only question remaining is the precise formulation.

Parenteral multi-vitamin preparations are used almost exclusively in hospitals for those patients who are unable to consume vitamins by mouth. The individual vitamins available for intravenous administration are effective when given in appropriate amounts. The idea behind the multi-vitamin preparations is to combine a number of different forms in one easy-to-administer vial.

However, according to the National Academy of Sciences-National Research Council, Folbesyn and the others in this class are inadequately formulated.

- **Brand Name: FORHISTAL LONTABS**
- **Manufacturer:** Ciba
- **Use:** Allergy
- **Dosage Form:** Time-release tablet
- **Administration:** Oral
- **Ingredients:** Dimethindene maleate 2.5 mg (antihistamine).

FORHISTAL is promoted for seasonal allergic nasal inflammation (hay fever), other nasal inflammatory conditions, allergic inflammations of the eye, certain allergic skin reactions, and as an adjunct to adrenalin therapy in severe systemic allergic (anaphylactic) reaction. Dimethindene maleate, like other antihistamines, is not effective in treating asthma or other serious allergic diseases. This is an example of an effective ingredient being formulated in a dubious manner; it is the time-release form that fails to meet adequately the standards of effectiveness. Forhistal is expensive, and its action can be uneven and unpredictable. At a fraction of the cost one could treat these allergic conditions with a single-entity generic antihistamine such as chlorpheniramine. Dimethindene can cause drowsiness, loss of coordination, mental inattention and dizziness. Identical drugs include: Triten Tab-In.

Also see Part II: Drugs for Cough, Cold and Allergy

- **Brand Name:** GEVIZOL
- **Manufacturer:** Saron
- **Use:** Central nervous system stimulation
- **Dosage Form:** Tablet / Elixir
- **Administration:** Oral / Oral
- **Ingredients:** Pentylenetetrazol (stimulant/analeptic); niacin (vitamin/vasodilator).

GEVIZOL is an irrational, ineffective mixture administered to enhance the mental and physical activity of elderly patients. The principal ingredient, pentylenetetrazol, is a central nervous system stimulant. However, there is no evidence to substantiate the efficacy of pentylenetetrazol, alone or in combination products, for the treatment of senility, mental depression, vertigo, or a disease of the inner ear (Meniere's). Niacin, taken in a much higher amount than is found in Gevizol, causes blood vessel dilation in the "blushing" areas. But it does nothing to lessen senility or mental and physical debility in the aged. Gevizol has been classified as ineffective by the FDA and, according to *AMA Drug Evaluations* (second edition, p. 379), has no proper place in modern medicine.

See similar drug RU-VERT, pg. 172

- **Brand Name: HYBEPHEN**
- **Manufacturer:** Beecham
- **Use:** Digestive disorders
- **Dosage Form:** Tablet /Elixir
- **Administration:** Oral / Oral
- **Ingredients:** Hyoscyamine sulfate, atropine sulfate, hyoscine hydrobromide (antispasmodic/antisecretories); phenobarbital (sedative); alcohol 16.5% (in elixir).

HYBEPHEN contains phenobarbital which can lead to psychological and physical addiction, and hyoscyamine, atropine and hyoscine which often cause blurring of vision, dryness of the mouth and throat, constipation and hesitancy of urination.

See similar drug DONNATAL, pg. 93
Also see Part II: Drugs for Digestive Disorders

- **Brand Name: HYCODAN**
- **Manufacturer:** Endo
- **Use:** Cough
- **Dosage Form:** Tablet /Syrup
- **Administration:** Oral / Oral
- **Ingredients:** Hydrocodone bitartrate (antitussive/narcotic); homatropine methylbromide (anticholinergic).

HYCODAN is sold for the symptomatic relief of cough. It is composed of an effective cough-suppressing component, hydrocodone, and a secretion-inhibiting component of questionable efficacy, homatropine. Homatropine may promote thickening of bronchial secretions and thus interfere with productive cough.

Productive cough, accompanied by a heavy discharge of mucus and phlegm (often seen in smokers with bronchial problems), is one of the body's ways of naturally ridding itself of secretions and guarding against infection. Dry cough can be treated with dextromethorphan (safer than the narcotic codeine), which is available without a prescription. Homatropine often causes blurring of vision, dryness of the mouth and throat, constipation and hesitancy of urination. Identical drugs include: Hydrocodone Syrup.

Also see Part II: Drugs for Cough, Cold and Allergy

- **Brand Name: HYDROCORTISONE-NEOMYCIN**
- **Manufacturer:** generic
- **Use:** Skin disorders
- **Dosage Form:** Ointment / Cream / Lotion
- **Administration:** Topical / Topical / Topical
- **Ingredients:** Neomycin sulfate (antibacterial); hydrocortisone (corticosteroid).

HYDROCORTISONE-NEOMYCIN

is a combination drug promoted for the treatment of a wide range of skin disorders and marketed by a number of generic firms. In general, hydrocortisone and other corticosteroids are not preferred for the treatment of skin infections. Moreover, antibiotics such as neomycin should not be used in the treatment of noninfectious skin problems. The use of corticosteroids for the treatment of skin infections may be dangerous because they can either mask the evidence of infection or cause the spreading of infections. Neomycin commonly causes skin rashes and can sensitize people to other more important antibiotics.

Also see Part II: Drugs Applied Directly to Skin, Eye or Ear

- **Brand Name: ILOTYCIN TOPICAL**
- **Manufacturer:** Dista(Lilly)
- **Use:** Skin infection, wound healing
- **Dosage Form:** Ointment
- **Administration:** Topical
- **Ingredients:** Erythromycin 1% (antibacterial).

ILOTYCIN TOPICAL is used in the treatment of certain skin infections caused by bacterial agents susceptible to erythromycin. It is also used to prevent infections in superficial wounds. However, there is insufficient evidence to demonstrate that Ilotycin is effective for these intended actions. The general use of topical antibacterials for skin wounds and infections is, at best, debatable. The topical administration of antibacterials should be avoided because of the danger of sensitization and the development of drug resistance, both of which could make erythromycin taken orally or by injection useless if a serious infection developed. Well-cleaned minor wounds and burns usually do very well by themselves, and if infection does set in, it is best to treat it with appropriate antibiotics given orally or by injection.

Also see Part II: Drugs Applied Directly to Skin, Eye or Ear

- Brand Name: **INDOGESIC**
- **Manufacturer:** Century
- **Use:** Pain relief
- **Dosage Form:** Tablet
- **Administration:** Oral
- **Ingredients:** Butabarbital sodium 10 mg (sedative); salicylamide 200 mg, acetaminophen 200 mg (analgesics).

INDOGESIC is a fixed-ratio combination drug used for the relief of pain associated with a variety of conditions. Of the three ingredients in Indogesic, only acetaminophen (as in Tylenol) is an analgesic (pain-reliever) of proven efficacy. Salicylamide, closely related to aspirin, has only weak analgesic properties and in effect adds very little to the acetaminophen. There are no controlled studies documenting the efficacy of sedatives, such as butabarbital sodium, in such mixtures. Indogesic is presently deemed ineffective as a fixed-combination by the FDA. If the use of a sedative is considered absolutely necessary, it should be administered separately according to the individual patient's requirements. But for the relief of mild to moderate pain associated with most conditions, either aspirin or acetaminophen alone is preferred. When taken regularly butabarbital can lead to psychological and physical addiction.

*See similar drug **BUTIGETIC**, pg. 65*

- **Brand Name: ISORDIL SUBLINGUAL**
- **Manufacturer:** Ives
- **Use:** Heart pain (angina pectoris)
- **Dosage Form:** Tablet
- **Administration:** Sublingual
- **Ingredients:** Isosorbide dinitrate 2.5 or 5 mg (coronary vasodilator).

ISORDIL SUBLINGUAL tablets, dissolved under the tongue, are sold and prescribed for the relief of chest pain due to acute anginal attacks, and for short-term prevention in those situations likely to provoke attacks, such as stress and physical exercise. When short-term relief or prevention of acute anginal pain is needed, the drug of choice is nitroglycerin tablets given under the tongue. Relief from an acute attack usually comes within one minute. Isosorbide lacks evidence of effectiveness for *treating* acute anginal attacks. Although FDA also presently classifies isosorbide as lacking evidence of effectiveness in *prevention* of anginal attacks, in one well-controlled study (*Chest* 73: 327-332, 1978) using very high doses (120 mg per day), the drug appeared to be effective for this purpose. Since it would take 48 of the 2.5 mg tablets a day or 24 of the 5 mg tablets to achieve a daily dose of 120 mg, it is unlikely that many people using this dosage form of isosorbide are getting a dose equal to that which was shown effective in the above study. Isosorbide is also being tested for use in heart failure with some studies showing favorable results; but, at this writing, it has not been approved for this indication. Identical drugs include: Iso-Bid, Isosorbide Dinitrate Sublingual, Isotrate Sublingual, Laserdil, Sorate-5, Sorate-2.5, Sorbitrate Sublingual.

Also see Part II: Drugs for Heart Pain

- **Brand Name: ISORDIL TEMBIDS**
- **Manufacturer:** Ives
- **Use:** Heart pain (angina pectoris)
- **Dosage Form:** Time-release tablet / Time-release capsule
- **Administration:** Oral / Oral
- **Ingredients:** Isosorbide dinitrate 40 mg, (coronary vasodilator).

ISORDIL TEMBIDS are promoted and prescribed for sustained reduction in the frequency and severity of transient heart pain (angina pectoris), a condition related to insufficient blood flow to the heart. In Part II, Drugs for Heart Pain, there is a discussion of one well-controlled study (*Chest* 73: 327-332, 1978) employing very high doses (120 mg per day) of Isordil capsules in which the drug appeared to be effective in preventing anginal attacks. Although the FDA says the drug lacks evidence of effectiveness, it is currently evaluating this study. However, most people using the 40 mg dosage form are getting less than 120 mg per day, the amount shown effective in the above study. Isordil is also being tested for use in heart failure with some studies showing favorable results. At this writing, however, it has not been approved for this indication. Identical drugs include: Iso-Bid, Isogard, Isosorbide Dinitrate, Isotrate Timecelles, Sorate-40, Sorbide T.D., Sorbitrate SA.

Also see Part II: Drugs for Heart Pain

- Brand Name: **ISORDIL TITRADOSE AND CHEWABLE TABLETS**
- **Manufacturer:** Ives
- **Use:** Heart pain (angina pectoris)
- **Dosage Form:** Tablet / Chewable tablet
- **Administration:** Oral / Oral
- **Ingredients:** Isosorbide dinitrate 5, 10 or 20 mg (coronary vasodilator).

ISORDIL TITRADOSE TABLETS,

swallowed whole, are prescribed for the prevention, control, and treatment of the transient pain of coronary artery disease (angina pectoris). However, this expensive and widely-used vasodilator has not been adequately proven effective in treating chest pain due to acute anginal attacks. Sublingual nitroglycerin (under the tongue), available in generic form and rated effective for short-term relief, is preferable. Although FDA presently classifies isosorbide as lacking evidence of effectiveness in *prevention* of anginal attacks, in one well-controlled study (*Chest* 73: 327-332, 1978) using very high doses, the drug appears to be effective for this purpose. But in 1979, about 90% of the prescriptions for Isordil Titradose were for the 5 or 10 mg dose, meaning someone would have to take twenty-four tablets of 5 mg each or twelve tablets of 10 mg each to achieve the dose of 120 mg per day shown effective in the above study. Isosorbide is also being tested for use in heart failure with some studies showing favorable results. At this writing, however, it has not been approved for this indication. Identical drugs include: Isosorbide Dinitrate, Onset-5, Onset-10, Sorbitrate, Isotrate, Sorate-5 Sorate-10, Sorbide-10, Vasotrate.

Also see Part II: Drugs for Heart Pain

- **Brand Name:** ISORDIL W/ PHENOBARBITAL
- **Manufacturer:** Ives
- **Use:** Heart pain (angina pectoris)
- **Dosage Form:** Tablet
- **Administration:** Oral
- **Ingredients:** Isosorbide dinitrate 10 mg (coronary vasodilator); phenobarbital 15 mg (sedative).

ISORDIL W/PHENOBARBITAL is sold
and used for the prevention, control and treatment of transient heart pain (angina pectoris). It is usually prescribed by doctors who believe that anxiety or emotional disturbances may be important factors in the clinical situation. However, as with the other oral nitrate-sedative combinations, the FDA has rated Isordil with Phenobarbital as "lacking substantial evidence of effectiveness."

According to the *AMA Drug Evaluations* (second edition, pg. 26) the use of combinations of this sort is unjustified. Long-acting nitrate vasodilators have not proved effective in preventing angina, and there is no convincing evidence that the added sedative has any therapeutic benefit. If occasional anxiety is a real problem in the anginal patient, a sedative and nitroglycerin (sublingual) should be administered separately. When taken regularly phenobarbital can lead to psychological and physical addiction.

Also see Part II: Drugs for Heart Pain

- **Brand Name: ISOVEX-100**
- **Manufacturer:** Medics
- **Use:** Blood vessel disease (head and limbs)
- **Dosage Form:** Capsule
- **Administration:** Oral
- **Ingredients:** Ethaverine hydrochloride 100 mg (vasodilator).

ISOVEX-100 is identical to the more widely used etha-verine product Ethatab in all respects except dosage form (capsule vs. tablet). Ethaverines are prescribed primarily to treat disorders arising from insufficient blood flow to the head and limbs and less frequently to treat pain due to lack of blood flow to the heart. These drugs are used widely among the elderly to treat some types of senility.

Ethaverine is a synthetic derivative of papaverine and both drugs have the same actions, although ethaverine is twice as potent. Cur-rently, there is no evidence that any ethaverine or papaverine product is effective for its recommended use; furthermore, there is strong evidence that these products cause liver damage in many people. (*New Eng J Med* 281:1333-35 and 1364-65, 1969). Identical drugs include: Cebral.

Also see Part II: Drugs for Circulatory Disorders of Head and Limbs

- **Brand Name: KINESED**
- **Manufacturer:** Stuart
- **Use:** Digestive disorders
- **Dosage Form:** Tablet
- **Administration:** Oral
- **Ingredients:** Hyoscyamine sulfate 0.1 mg, atropine sulfate 0.02 mg, hyoscine hydrobromide 0.007 mg (antispasmodic/antisecretories); phenobarbital 16 mg (sedative).

KINESED is prescribed as adjunctive therapy for patients with stomach ulcer, irritable bowel syndrome or other gastrointes-tinal disorders. However, this product lacks sufficient evidence of efficacy as a fixed-combination.

Kinesed is very similar to Donnatal in both content and dosage amount. There is no evidence that antispasmodic/antisecretory drugs promote the healing of stomach ulcer, prevent its recurrence or directly improve organic bowel disease. Fixed-combinations such as Kinesed and Donnatal remain of unproven effectiveness and highly questionable value, especially in light of the fact that the amounts of the antispasmodic/antisecretory agents included are so small. In addition, when taken regularly, phenobarbital can lead to psychological and physical addiction. Hyoscyamine, atropine and hyoscine often cause blurring of vision, dryness of the mouth and throat, constipation and hesitancy of urination.

Also see Part II: Drugs for Digestive Disorders

- **Brand Name: LAPAV**
- **Manufacturer:** Amfre-Grant
- **Use:** Blood vessel disease (head and limbs)
- **Dosage Form:** Elixir
- **Administration:** Oral
- **Ingredients:** Papaverine hydrochloride 100 mg per 15 ml (vasodilator); alcohol 10%.

LAPAV is the only liquid papaverine product in this book and, like other papaverines, it is prescribed for treating disorders due to insufficient blood flow to the head and limbs and pain due to insufficient blood flow to the heart. Papaverines are used predominantly by the elderly.

There is no evidence that papaverine in any dosage form works for its recommended uses. In addition, there is strong evidence that papaverines can cause liver damage in many people (*New Eng J Med* 281: 1333-35 and 1364-65, 1969).

See similar drug PAPAVERINE, pg. 143

Also see Part II: Drugs for Circulatory Disorders of Head and Limbs

- **Brand Name: LEVSIN W/ PHENOBARBITAL**
- **Manufacturer:** Kremers-Urban
- **Use:** Digestive disorders
- **Dosage Form:** Tablet /Elixir
- **Administration:** Oral/ Oral
- **Ingredients:** Hyoscyamine sulfate (antispasmodic/ antisecretory); phenobarbital (sedative).

LEVSIN W/PHENOBARBITAL is a fixed-combination product used for a variety of conditions whenever the actions of an antispasmodic/antisecretory drug (these drugs act to suppress certain secretions such as stomach acid) and a sedative are desired. This particular product is prescribed primarily for a wide variety of digestive disorders, including peptic ulcer and the irritable bowel syndrome. It is also promoted to control symptoms of Parkinsonism.

Levsin with Phenobarbital suffers from all of the disadvantages of a fixed-ratio combination. If sedatives are truly deemed appropriate by one's doctor, they should be administered separately and adjusted to one's specific needs. When taken regularly, phenobarbital can lead to psychological and physical addiction. Hyoscyamine often causes blurring of vision, dryness of the mouth and throat, constipation and hesitancy of urination. Identical drugs include: Anaspaz PB.

See similar drug DONNATAL, pg. 93

Also see Part II: Drugs for Digestive Disorders

- **Brand Name: LIBRAX**
- **Manufacturer:** Roche
- **Use:** Digestive disorders
- **Dosage Form:** Tablet
- **Administration:** Oral
- **Ingredients:** Clidinium bromide 2.5 mg (antispasmodic/ antisecretory); chlordiazepoxide hydrochloride 5 mg (tranquilizer).

LIBRAX is advertised as "a useful adjunct for relief of irritable bowel syndrome because it combats both excessive anxiety and associated G.I. [gastrointestinal] symptoms." There is no convincing evidence that Librax is an effective combination. If a patient suffers from an ulcer and, because of this, movement of food through the stomach should be slowed, an effective dose of atropine may be used. If the cause of the G.I. disorders is anxiety, a sedative which is suited to the individual's needs may be prescribed separately. Clidinium often causes blurring of vision, dryness of the mouth and throat, constipation and hesitancy of urination. Identical drugs include: Clipoxide, Lidinium.

WARNING: The use of minor tranquilizers such as meprobamate (Miltown), chlordiazepoxide (Librium), diazepam (Valium) or similar drugs during pregnancy should be avoided because of increased risk of damage to the developing fetus. One must consider the possibility of pregnancy when beginning minor tranquilizer therapy. In the case of combination drugs such as Librax, use at any time is unwarranted.

Also see Part II: Drugs for Digestive Disorders

- Brand Name: **LIDOSPORIN OTIC**
- **Manufacturer:** Burroughs Wellcome
- **Use:** Ear infection
- **Dosage Form:** Solution
- **Administration:** Ear
- **Ingredients:** Polymyxin B sulfate 10,000 u (antibacterial); lidocaine hydrochloride 5% (anesthetic).

LIDOSPORIN OTIC solution is prescribed for the treatment of external ear infections. This product combines a broad-spectrum antibiotic (polymyxin) with a local anesthetic (lidocaine).

There are several shortcomings of the use of local anesthetics in ear drop solutions. They may produce allergy; they can mask symptoms of serious ear disorders; and their efficacy is unestablished. Topically-applied antibiotics for the treatment of ear infections are also of questionable effectiveness. If the infection is serious, antibiotics should be given orally or by injection after the causal agent has been identified by culture; less serious external ear infections are often self-limited.

Also see Part II: Drugs Applied Directly to Skin, Eye or Ear

- **Brand Name: LUFTODIL**
- **Manufacturer:** Wallace
- **Use:** Asthma, respiratory disorders
- **Dosage Form:** Tablet
- **Administration:** Oral
- **Ingredients:** Theophylline 100 mg, ephedrine hydrochloride 24 mg (bronchodilators); phenobarbital 16 mg (sedative); guaifenesin 200 mg (expectorant).

LUFTODIL is a polypharmaceutical product prescribed for the prevention and symptomatic treatment of asthma and similar respiratory problems, such as emphysema.

Theophylline, at the proper individualized dose, effectively relaxes and dilates the breathing passages, and can make breathing easier in some cases of asthma. The dose in this product may not be effective for many people. Ephedrine, an adrenalin-like drug that also dilates breathing passages, commonly loses its effectiveness when given regularly. It can also cause or aggravate high blood pressure. There is no convincing evidence that sedatives like phenobarbital contribute any significant effect towards lessening asthma. In fact, they may be harmful since they can decrease the impulse to breathe. In addition, there is no evidence of the clinical efficacy of the expectorant (phlegm-loosening agent) guaifenesin in asthma products.

- **Brand Name: LUFYLLIN-EPG**
- **Manufacturer:** Wallace
- **Use:** Asthma, respiratory disorders
- **Dosage Form:** Tablet /Elixir
- **Administration:** Oral / Oral
- **Ingredients:** Ephedrine hydrochloride, dyphylline (bronchodilators); phenobarbital (sedative); guaifenesin (expectorant); alcohol 5.5% (in elixir).

LUFYLLIN-EPG is a multi-ingredient product administered for the prevention and symptomatic treatment of asthma and similar respiratory conditions where wheezing and constricted ("tight") air passages are significant problems. It has been rated ineffective as a fixed-combination by the FDA.

There is also no satisfactory evidence that the expectorant (phlegm-loosening agent) guaifenesin is efficacious in asthma products such as Lufyllin-EPG.

Ephedrine can cause or aggravate high blood pressure and commonly loses its effectiveness when used regularly. Dyphylline can be effective for treating asthma if used at the proper individualized dose. The dose in this product may not be effective for many people. There is no clinical evidence that phenobarbital is effective in the treatment of asthma and phenobarbital can be psychologically and physically addicting if used regularly.

See similar drugs, AMESEC & LUFTODIL, pg. 47, 114

- Brand Name: **MANNITOL HEXANITRATE**
- **Manufacturer:** generic
- **Use:** Heart pain (angina pectoris)
- **Dosage Form:** Tablet
- **Administration:** Oral
- **Ingredients:** Mannitol hexanitrate (coronary vasodilator).

MANNITOL HEXANITRATE is an organic nitrate blood vessel dilator used to reduce in frequency and severity the pain associated with angina (transient heart pain). Although mannitol hexanitrate in its various forms does produce dilation of the coronary arteries, there is no convincing evidence that its daily ingestion will successfully prevent angina or lessen the frequency and severity of attacks.

Also see Part II: Drugs for Heart Pain

- Brand Name: **MANNITOL HEXANITRATE W/PHENOBARBITAL**
- **Manufacturer:** generic
- **Use:** Heart pain (angina pectoris)
- **Dosage Form:** Tablet
- **Administration:** Oral
- **Ingredients:** Mannitol hexanitrate 32 mg (coronary vasodilator); phenobarbital 16 mg (sedative).

MANNITOL HEXANITRATE W/ PHENOBARBITAL is an oral nitrate blood vessel dilating agent administered to reduce in frequency and severity the

transient pain due to coronary artery disease (angina pectoris). However, there is no convincing evidence that longterm, daily consump-
tion of this drug is of value in the prevention and management of the
anginal syndrome. Mannitol hexanitrate with phenobarbital is usually prescribed when the physician believes anxiety or emotional disturbances may be important factors. Although sedatives may be useful in some patients with angina pectoris, they should be administered
alone and not as part of combination regimens such as mannitol
hexanitrate with phenobarbital. When taken regularly, phenobarbital can lead to psychological and physical addiction.

Also see Part II: Drugs for Heart Pain

- Brand Name: **MARAX** and **MARAX DF**
- **Manufacturer:** Roerig
- **Use:** Asthma, respiratory disorders
- **Dosage Form:** Tablet /Syrup
- **Administration:** Oral / Oral
- **Ingredients:** Ephedrine sulfate, theophylline (bronchodilators);
  hydroxyzine hydrochloride (sedative); alcohol 5% (in syrup).

MARAX is prescribed for treatment of asthma and related respiratory problems. The ingredient theophylline is effective for these
uses but is present in insufficient amounts (130 mg per tablet or 20 ml
of syrup) for many asthma patients. Ephedrine, an adrenalin-like
drug, dilates air passages but often loses its effectiveness when taken
on a prolonged basis. Moreover, ephedrine may cause or aggravate
high blood pressure. Hydroxyzine, a sedative, has been shown in
clinical studies to produce no benefit in this combination. If your doctor believes that a sedative is called for, he/she should prescribe it
in an amount adjusted to your individual need.

   In general, single ingredient generic drugs like theophylline or
aminophylline, at the proper individualized dose, are preferred for
asthma treatment. The unnecessary additional ingredients in products like Marax add to the cost and increase the risk of unwanted and
sometimes dangerous side effects. Identical drugs include: Asmino-
rel Improved, E.T.H. Compound, Hydrophed, Theophozine, Theo-
zine.

See similar drug AMESEC, pg. 47

- **Brand Name: MARPLAN**
- **Manufacturer:** Roche
- **Use:** Anti-depressant
- **Dosage Form:** Tablet
- **Administration:** Oral
- **Ingredients:** Isocarboxazid (monoamine oxidase inhibitor)

MARPLAN is recommended by the manufacturer for use in the treatment of depressed patients who fail to improve with tricyclic anti-depressants or shock therapy (ECT)* Like other drugs in its class (monoamine oxidase inhibitors), isocarboxazid is less effective and more dangerous than the tricyclic compounds. The FDA has rated this drug as ineffective.

WARNING: Fatal reactions to this drug (hypertensive crises) can occur when it is used with drugs such as amphetamines or with cheese, beer, wine and other foods.

---

*ECT is a potentially beneficial means of therapy for selected patients under certain circumstances. However, the FDA's current standards for electroshock machines are inadequate so it may be being used inappropriately or improperly.

- **Brand Name: MEDROL ENPAK**
- **Manufacturer:** Upjohn
- **Use:** Intestinal disorders
- **Dosage Form:** Suppository
- **Administration:** Rectal
- **Ingredients:** Methylprednisolone acetate 40 mg (corticosteroid).

MEDROL ENPAK is used as a retention enema for the adjunctive treatment of several inflammatory diseases of the rectum and sigmoid colon, ulcerative colitis in particular. This product is also sometimes used to treat inflammation of the prostate caused by irradiation. It has been rated by the FDA as "less than effective" for its labeled indications. According to the *AMA Drug Evaluations* (third edition, p. 1065), "less than 50 percent of patients experience a relief of symptoms, and those who are most likely to respond cannot be predicted in advance."

There are a number of potential adverse reactions associated with corticosteroid therapy. Substantial amounts of the drug are absorbed from the inflamed intestine. Corticosteroids may also mask some signs of infection, and can decrease the body's resistance to infection.

- **Brand Name: MEPERGAN FORTIS**
- **Manufacturer:** Wyeth
- **Use:** Moderate to severe pain relief
- **Dosage Form:** Capsule
- **Administration:** Oral
- **Ingredients:** Promethazine hydrochloride 25 mg (antihistamine/sedative); meperidine hydrochloride 50 mg (narcotic analgesic).

MEPERGAN FORTIS is prescribed for the relief of moderate to severe pain related to a wide variety of conditions. The manufacturer's claims that the promethazine ingredient adds to the pain-relieving. effect of meperidine, a narcotic, have not been confirmed. Mepergan is sometimes used as a sedative before surgery, but the FDA has never rated it effective as a fixed-combination. The question is whether this particular formulation has any distinct advantage over meperidine alone. The FDA has concluded it does not, and the *AMA Drug Evaluations* (second edition, pg. 260) states that "in final analysis, there is insufficient evidence to indicate that Mepergan has any advantage over meperidine alone for analgesia."

Promethazine is sometimes used to treat nausea and vomiting. Because it is an antihistamine, it is found in certain cough and cold preparations as well (e.g. Phenergan Expectorant). Promethazine can cause drowsiness, loss of coordination, mental inattention and dizziness. Although occurring rarely, blood disorders have been associated with prolonged use of promethazine. In the case of Mepergan Fortis, the addition of promethazine does not provide benefit or increase pain relief, while it does add unnecessary side effects.

See similar drug SYNALGOS, pg. 174, for discussion of unnecessary ingredients in fixed-combination pain relievers.

- **Brand Name: METIMYD**
- **Manufacturer:** Schering
- **Use:** Eye disorders
- **Dosage Form:** Suspension / Ointment
- **Administration:** Eye   /   Eye
- **Ingredients:** Sodium sulfacetamide 10% (antibacterial); prednisolone acetate 0.5% (corticosteroid).

METIMYD is used for the treatment of inflammation and allergic reaction of the eyelids and the eye. This drug and similar fixed-combinations are not appropriate for these disorders, as prednisolone may actually worsen some eye infections, according to *AMA Drug Evaluations* (third edition, pg. 971). Identical drugs include: Ophtha P/S Ophthalmic Drops, Vasocidin Ointment.

Also see Part II: Drugs Applied Directly to Skin, Eye or Ear

- **Brand Name: METRAZOL**
- **Manufacturer:** Knoll
- **Use:** Central nervous system stimulation
- **Dosage Form:** Tablet / Elixir
- **Administration:** Oral / Oral
- **Ingredients:** Pentylenetetrazol (stimulant/analeptic); alcohol 15% (in elixir).

METRAZOL, in its tablet and elixir forms, is administered to enhance the mental and physical activity of elderly patients. Pentylenetetrazol is a central nervous system stimulant used in the past to stimulate breathing. There is nothing to justify its use in the treatment of senility, mental depression, vertigo, or a disease of the inner ear (Meniere's). The FDA has rated this product as ineffective, and the *AMA Drug Evaluations* (second edition, pg. 379) states that pentylenetetrazol-containing drugs have no valid place in modern medicine. Identical drugs include: Nelex-100, Nioric.

See similar drug RU-VERT, pg. 172

- **Brand Name: MIGRAL**
- **Manufacturer:** Burroughs Wellcome
- **Use:** Migraine headache
- **Dosage Form:** Tablet
- **Administration:** Oral
- **Ingredients:** Ergotamine tartrate 1 mg (blood vessel constrictor); cyclizine 25 mg (antihistamine); caffeine 50 mg (stimulant).

MIGRAL is used to treat vascular headache, including migraine. The FDA has proposed to withdraw approval of this product because Migral has not proved to be an effective drug combination. Although ergotamine tartrate is the drug of choice for migraine headache episodes, the daily use of this drug as a preventive measure is inadvisable. Side effects of ergotamine, especially with overdosage, include a sensation of cold hands and feet with numbness. No studies have shown conclusively that cyclizine (an antihistamine) adds any benefit. In addition, cyclizine can cause drowsiness, loss of coordination, mental inattention and dizziness. Caffeine adds no beneficial effect to that of ergotamine. Ergotamine alone is available generically at a much lower cost.

- **Brand Name: MILTRATE**
- **Manufacturer:** Wallace
- **Use:** Heart pain (angina pectoris)
- **Dosage Form:** Tablet
- **Administration:** Oral
- **Ingredients:** Pentaerythritol tetranitrate 10 or 20 mg (coronary vasodilator); meprobamate 200 mg (sedative).

MILTRATE is a fixed-combination product sold and used in the treatment and prevention of transient heart pain (angina pectoris). It is also employed to reduce emotional stress in angina patients because it contains the sedative meprobamate. The FDA has reclassified this combination as ineffective. Although sedatives may be useful to reduce reactions to emotional stress in certain angina patients, they should be prescribed separately, if truly needed. Oral nitrates, such as pentaerythritol tetranitrate, have not been shown to prevent or lessen angina. Identical drugs include: Equanitrate.

WARNING: The use of minor tranquilizers such as meprobamate (Miltown), chlordiazepoxide (Librium), diazepam (Valium)
or similar drugs during pregnancy should be avoided because of increased risk of damage to the developing fetus. One must consider
the possibility of pregnancy when beginning minor tranquilizer
therapy. In the case of combination drugs such as Miltrate, use at
any time is unwarranted.

Also see Part II: Drugs for Heart Pain

- Brand Name: **M.V.I. INJECTION**
- **Manufacturer:** USV
- **Use:** Vitamin deficiency
- **Dosage Form:** Solution
- **Administration:** Intravenous
- **Ingredients:** Vitamins A, D, E, C, B-1, B-2, niacinamide,
B-6, pantheol (multi-vitamins).

M.V.I. is used to prevent or to treat vitamin deficiencies in certain diseases after surgery. As presently formulated, this multi-
vitamin preparation has been ruled ineffective by the FDA. This is
entirely a matter of ascertaining the proper proportions of each
ingredient in the mixture. The individual ingredients are not ineffective per se, but when combined in products such as M.V.I. they fail to
satisfy the requirements for effectiveness.

Intravenous multi-vitamin products are used almost exclusively in
hospitals for those patients who are unable to take vitamin pills or
food. Individual vitamins, available for intravenous administration,
are effective when given in appropriate amounts.

See similar drug FOLBESYN, pg. 102

- **Brand Name: MYCOLOG**
- **Manufacturer:** Squibb
- **Use:** Skin disorders, infection
- **Dosage Form:** Cream / Ointment
- **Administration:** Topical / Topical
- **Ingredients:** Neomycin sulfate .25%, gramicidin 0.25 mg (antibacterials); triamcinolone acetonide .1% (corticosteroid); nystatin 100,000 u (antifungal) per gram.

MYCOLOG is a combination drug used for various skin disorders and skin infections. It is composed of two antibacterials, neomycin and gramicidin; an antifungal drug, nystatin; and a steroid (anti-inflammatory drug), triamcinolone. There is inadequate evidence that this combination is effective in promoting wound healing or resolving skin infections. For yeast infections of skin, nystatin is useful, but it should be given alone. The use of corticosteroids for the treatment of skin infections may be dangerous because they can either mask the evidence of infection or cause the spreading of infections. Neomycin commonly causes skin rashes and can sensitize people to other more important antibiotics.

Also see Part II: Drugs Applied Directly to Skin, Eye or Ear

- **Brand Name: MYSTECLIN F**
- **Manufacturer:** Squibb
- **Use:** Bacterial and fungal infection
- **Dosage Form:** Capsule / Syrup
- **Administration:** Oral / Oral
- **Ingredients:** Tetracycline (antibacterial); amphotericin B (antifungal).

MYSTECLIN F is a mixture which contains tetracycline phosphate, a broad-spectrum antibacterial agent, in combination with the antifungal agent amphotericin B, and is designed to prevent the overgrowth of intestinal fungi once the bacterial infection is eradicated. The alleged rationale behind this sort of formulation is that tetracycline often alters the normal bacteria in the intestine, thereby allowing a proliferation or "overgrowth" of the yeast Candida albicans. Because amphotericin B in appropriate amounts is effective in combating yeast growth, manufacturers claim it should prevent such an overgrowth by being mixed with tetracycline in "prophylactic amounts" (50 mg/tablet). The rationale for use of this fixed-combination is weak. Intestinal yeast infection does not occur very often and there is no clinical evidence that the routine "preventive" administration of an antifungal agent reduces its incidence (*AMA Drug Evaluations,* second edition, pg. 597).

With regard to antibiotic therapy, two general rules apply. First, the use of an antibiotic to prevent an infection from ever occurring is rarely necessary, except perhaps during certain surgical procedures or in patients with a history of rheumatic fever. In the case of Mysteclin F, the amount of antifungal agent used is below the therapeutic quantity required to block most yeast overgrowth anyway. Second, if an antifungal drug is needed to treat intestinal yeast infection in a patient receiving an antibacterial agent, it is preferable to give the two drugs separately. In this way, the doctor can adjust the amounts according to the patient's specific needs, and can be sure that each drug is given at the optimal therapeutic level.

A report issued by a scientific panel of the National Academy of Sciences-National Research Council (NAS-NRC) states that, "It is preferable, in the Panel's opinion, to prescribe antifungal drugs where clinically indicated, rather than to use them indiscriminately as prophylaxis against an uncommon clinical entity during therapy with tetracycline and other antibiotics."

When an antifungal agent is called for, nystatin is preferred because it has fewer side effects than amphotericin B and costs less, although both drugs can cause nausea and vomiting when given orally.

Mysteclin F is a classic example of a mixture of two relatively inexpensive drugs (if purchased in single-entity generic forms) to yield a brand name product that provides no real additional therapeutic benefit, but is extremely expensive and exposes the patient to undesired potential side effects.

- **Brand Name: NATURETIN WITH K**
- **Manufacturer:** Squibb
- **Use:** High blood pressure and fluid retention
- **Dosage Form:** Tablet
- **Administration:** Oral
- **Ingredients:** Bendroflumethiazide 2.5 or 5 mg (diuretic); potassium chloride 500 mg (salt).

NATURETIN WITH K is used to treat fluid retention and swelling (edema), which can be caused by heart or kidney failure, liver disease or various drugs. The drug is also used to treat high blood pressure. However, the FDA has found this fixed-combination product to be of unproven safety and efficacy.

The use of a diuretic for high blood pressure and edema is reasonable. Since most diuretics cause a loss of potassium, an important mineral, oral potassium must often be taken as well. Naturetin with K (potassium), however, contains a fixed, small amount of potassium, not likely to be enough to make up for the loss. The combination may thus create a false sense of security that could allow potassium deficiency to develop. In addition, potassium salts found in tablet or capsule form have been blamed for causing serious intestinal ulcers, and some people may not need potassium or may even be harmed by it.

Potassium should therefore be given separately as a dietary supplement or as a solution (safer, less expensive forms), and tailored to each person's individual needs. For reasons of safety and effectiveness as well as cost, Naturetin with K and similar products should be avoided.

- Brand Name: **NEO-CORT-DOME**
- **Manufacturer:** Dome
- **Use:** Skin disorders
- **Dosage Form:** Cream / Lotion
- **Administration:** Topical / Topical
- **Ingredients:** Neomycin sulfate .5% (antibacterial); hydrocortisone acetate .25, .5 or 1% (corticosteroid).

NEO-CORT-DOME is used for the relief of inflammatory skin disorders complicated by bacterial infections. The use of corticosteroids for the treatment of skin infections may be dangerous because they can either mask the evidence of infection or cause the spreading of infections. Neomycin commonly causes skin rashes and can sensitize people to other more important antibiotics.

Also see Part II: Drugs Applied Directly to Skin, Eye or Ear

- Brand Name: **NEO-CORTEF OPHTHALMIC**
- **Manufacturer:** Upjohn
- **Use:** Eye infection, allergy
- **Dosage Form:** Ointment / Suspension
- **Administration:** Eye / Eye
- **Ingredients:** Neomycin sulfate .5% (antibacterial); hydrocortisone acetate .5 or 1.5% (corticosteroid).

NEO-CORTEF OPHTHALMIC is used
in the treatment of various eye and eyelid infections of bacterial and allergic origin. The use of corticosteroids for the treatment of eye infections may be dangerous because they can either mask the evidence of infection or cause the spreading of infections. Neomycin commonly causes skin rashes and can sensitize people to other more important antibiotics. Identical drugs include: Ak-Neo-Cort, Cor-Oticin, Ophthel (Improved).

Also see Part II: Drugs Applied Directly to Skin, Eye or Ear

- Brand Name: **NEO-CORTEF TOPICAL**
- **Manufacturer:** Upjohn
- **Use:** Skin disorders
- **Dosage Form:** Cream /Ointment/ Lotion
- **Administration:** Topical/ Topical /Topical
- **Ingredients:** Neomycin sulfate .5% (antibacterial); hydrocortisone acetate .5, 1, or 2.5% (corticosteroid).

NEO-CORTEF TOPICAL is used to treat
various skin disorders complicated by infections. A mixture of an antibiotic and a corticosteroid, Neo-Cortef is claimed by the manufacturer to be superior to either ingredient alone for the treatment of infected eczema. There is no convincing evidence, however, that antibiotics applied to the skin are useful against infection, and neomycin commonly causes skin rashes and can sensitize people to other more important antibiotics. The use of corticosteroids for the treatment of skin infections may be dangerous because they can either mask the evidence of infection or cause the spreading of infections.

Also see Part II: Drugs Applied Directly to Skin, Eye or Ear

- **Brand Name:** **NEO-DECADRON OPHTHALMIC**
- **Manufacturer:** Merck Sharp & Dohme
- **Use:** Eye infection
- **Dosage Form:** Solution / Ointment
- **Administration:** Eye / Eye
- **Ingredients:** Neomycin sulfate .5% (antibacterial); dexamethasone sodium phosphate .05 or .1% (corticosteroid).

NEO-DECADRON OPHTHALMIC is used to treat various eye and eyelid infections of bacterial and allergic origin. There has been no persuasive proof of its efficacy as a fixed-combination in treating eye infections.

In general, combination products containing corticosteroids and antibiotics are "not recommended for the topical [external] treatment of ocular [eye] infections," according to the *AMA Drug Evaluations* (first edition, pg. 526). The use of corticosteroids for the treatment of eye infections may be dangerous because they can either mask the evidence of infection or cause the spreading of infections. Neomycin commonly causes skin rashes and can sensitize people to other more important antibiotics.

See similar drug: NEO-CORTEF OPHTHALMIC, pg. 124

Also see Part II: Drugs Applied Directly to Skin, Eye or Ear

- **Brand Name:** **NEO-DECADRON TOPICAL**
- **Manufacturer:** Merck Sharp & Dohme
- **Use:** Skin disorders
- **Dosage Form:** Cream
- **Administration:** Topical
- **Ingredients:** Neomycin sulfate .5% (antibacterial); dexamethasone sodium phosphate .1% (corticosteroid).

NEO-DECADRON TOPICAL is a fixed-combination product used for the relief and management of various skin disorders complicated by infections. It is also used to promote healing or prevent infections of wounds. Topical antibiotics, particularly neomycin, have little usefulness, and furthermore neomycin commonly causes skin rashes and can sensitize people to other more important antibiotics. The use of corticosteroids for the treatment of skin infections may be dangerous because they can either mask the evidence of infection or cause the spreading of infections.

See similar drug NEO-CORT-DOME, pg. 124

Also see Part II: Drugs Applied Directly to Skin, Eye or Ear

- Brand Name: **NEO-DELTA-CORTEF OPHTHALMIC**
- **Manufacturer:** Upjohn
- **Use:** Eye infection
- **Dosage Form:** Drops   Ointment
- **Administration:** Eye   Eye
- **Ingredients:** Neomycin sulfate (antibacterial); prednisolone acetate (corticosteroid).

NEO-DELTA-CORTEF
OPHTHALMIC is an antibiotic-corticosteroid combination product used to treat various eye and eyelid infections of bacterial and allergic origin. The use of corticosteroids for the treatment of eye infections may be dangerous because they can either mask the evidence of infection or cause the spreading of infections. Neomycin commonly causes skin rashes and can sensitize people to other more important antibiotics.

See similar drug NEO-DECADRON OPHTHALMIC, pg. 126

Also see Part II: Drugs Applied Directly to Skin, Eye or Ear

- **Brand Name: NEO-DELTA-CORTEF TOPICAL**
- **Manufacturer:** Upjohn
- **Use:** Skin disorders
- **Dosage Form:** Ointment
- **Administration:** Topical
- **Ingredients:** Neomycin sulfate .5% (antibacterial); prednisolone acetate .5% (corticosteroid).

NEO-DELTA-CORTEF TOPICAL is a fixed-combination product used to treat various skin disorders complicated by infections. This mixture of a corticosteroid, prednisolone, with the antibiotic neomycin is entirely irrational. The use of corticosteroids for the treatment of skin infections may be dangerous because they can either mask the evidence of infection or cause the spreading of infections. Neomycin commonly causes skin rashes and can sensitize people to other more important antibiotics.

Also see Part II: Drugs Applied Directly to Skin, Eye or Ear

- **Brand Name: NEO-HYDELTRASOL OPHTHALMIC**
- **Manufacturer:** Merck Sharp & Dohme
- **Use:** Eye infection, inflammation
- **Dosage Form:** Solution / Ointment
- **Administration:** Eye / Eye
- **Ingredients:** Neomycin sulfate 0.5% (antibacterial); prednisolone sodium phosphate 0.25 or 0.5% (corticosteroid).

NEO-HYDELTRASOL OPHTHALMIC is an antibiotic-corticosteroid combination used in the treatment of various eye and eyelid infections of bacterial and allergic origin. The use of corticosteroids for the treatment of eye infections may be dangerous because they can either mask the evidence of infection or cause the spreading of infections. Neomycin commonly causes skin rashes and can sensitize people to other more important antibiotics.

See similar drug METIMYD, pg. 119

Also see Part II: Drugs Applied Directly to Skin, Eye or Ear

- **Brand Name: NEO-MEDROL ACETATE**
- **Manufacturer:** Upjohn
- **Use:** Skin disorders
- **Dosage Form:** Cream
- **Administration:** Topical
- **Ingredients:** Neomycin sulfate .5% (antibacterial); methylprednisolone acetate .25 or 1% (corticosteroid).

NEO-MEDROL ACETATE is one of many antibiotic-corticosteroid topical preparations used to treat various skin disorders complicated by infections. This type of mixture of a corticosteroid such as methylprednisolone with the antibiotic neomycin is irrational. The use of corticosteroids for the treatment of skin infections may be dangerous because they can either mask the evidence of infection or cause the spreading of infections. Neomycin commonly causes skin rashes and can sensitize people to other more important antibiotics.

Also see Part II: Drugs Applied Directly to Skin, Eye or Ear

- **Brand Name: NEO-MEDROL OPHTHALMIC**
- **Manufacturer:** Upjohn
- **Use:** Eye infection, inflammation
- **Dosage Form:** Ointment
- **Administration:** Eye
- **Ingredients:** Neomycin sulfate 0.5% (antibacterial); methylprednisolone 0.1% (corticosteroid).

NEO-MEDROL OPHTHALMIC is used in the treatment of various eye and eyelid infections and allergies. It is a fixed-dose polypharmaceutical containing a corticosteroid along with the antibiotic neomycin. The use of corticosteroids for the treatment of skin infections may be dangerous because they can either mask the evidence of infection or cause the spreading of infections. Neomycin commonly causes skin rashes and can sensitize people to other more important antibiotics.

See similar drug CORTISPORIN OPHTHALMIC, pg. 80

Also see Part II: Drugs Applied Directly to Skin, Eye or Ear.

- **Brand Name: NEO-OXYLONE**
- **Manufacturer:** Upjohn
- **Use:** Skin disorders
- **Dosage Form:** Ointment
- **Administration:** Topical
- **Ingredients:** Neomycin sulfate 0.5% (antibacterial); fluorometholone 0.025% (corticosteroid).

NEO-OXYLONE is used to treat allergic and inflammatory skin disorders complicated by infection. The use of corticosteroids for the treatment of skin infections may be dangerous because they can either mask the evidence of infection or cause the spreading of infections. Neomycin commonly causes skin rashes and can sensitize people to other more important antibiotics. Antibacterial agents should never be used for non-infectious skin problems.

Also see Part II: Drugs Applied Directly to Skin, Eye or Ear

- **Brand Name: NEOPAVRIN FORTE**
- **Manufacturer:** Savage
- **Use:** Blood vessel disease (head and limbs)
- **Dosage Form:** Tablet
- **Administration:** Oral
- **Ingredients:** Ethaverine hydrochloride 90 mg (vasodilator).

NEOPAVRIN FORTE is prescribed for disorders resulting from insufficient blood flow to the head and limbs. Like all ethaverine and papaverine products, there is no evidence that Neopavrin Forte works, and there is strong evidence that ethaverine can cause liver damage in many people (*New Eng J Med* 281:1333-35 and 1364-65, 1969).

See similar drug ETHATAB, pg. 100

Also see Part II: Drugs for Circulatory Disorders of Head and Limbs

- **Brand Name: NEOSONE**
- **Manufacturer:** Upjohn
- **Use:** Eye infection
- **Dosage Form:** Ointment
- **Administration:** Eye
- **Ingredients:** Neomycin sulfate 0.5% (antibacterial); cortisone acetate 1.5% (corticosteroid).

NEOSONE is one of numerous available antibiotic-corticosteroid combinations used to treat various eye and eyelid conditions of allergic and infectious origin. The use of corticosteroids for the treatment of eye infections may be dangerous because they can either mask the evidence of infection or cause the spreading of infections. Neomycin commonly causes skin rashes and can sensitize people to other more important antibiotics.

See similar drug NEO-CORTEF OPHTHALMIC, pg. 124

Also see Part II: Drugs Applied Directly to Skin, Eye or Ear

- **Brand Name: NEOSPORIN**
- **Manufacturer:** Burroughs Wellcome
- **Use:** Skin infection, wound healing
- **Dosage Form:** Aerosol / Powder / Ointment
- **Administration:** Topical / Topical / Topical
- **Ingredients:** Neomycin sulfate, polymyxin B sulfate, zinc bacitracin (antibacterials).

NEOSPORIN, found in aerosol spray, powder and ointment form, is an antibiotic combination used to treat a wide variety of skin infections. Neosporin is also used to prevent infection in burns or broken skin.

The drug has a broad spectrum of antibacterial activity. However, the use of topical antibiotics for wounds and infections is, at best, debatable. There is no satisfactory clinical evidence that they promote healing or prevent infections. If infections are present in wounds, and antibiotics are required, they should be given orally or by injection. Uninfected, well-cleaned wounds usually do well by themselves.

In the ads, the manufacturer touts Neosporin as "highly recommended . . . and for good reasons." The FDA disagrees. In its recent review of over-the-counter medications, the FDA found all topical antibiotic products containing neomycin as unproven in efficacy. Neomycin commonly causes skin rashes and can sensitize people to other more important antibiotics. Identical drugs include: Neo-Polycin.

Also see Part II: Drugs Applied Directly to Skin, Eye or Ear

- Brand Name: **NEOSPORIN-G**
- **Manufacturer:** Burroughs Wellcome
- **Use:** Skin disorders, wound healing
- **Dosage Form:** Cream
- **Administration:** Topical
- **Ingredients:** Neomycin sulfate 5 mg, gramicidin 0.25 mg, polymyxin B sulfate 10,000 u (antibacterials) per gram.

NEOSPORIN-G, similar in composition to the over-the-counter product Neosporin, is offered only by prescription. Neomycin commonly causes skin rashes and can sensitize people to other more important antibiotics.

See similar drug NEOSPORIN, pg. 131

Also see Part II: Drugs Applied Directly to Skin, Eye or Ear

- Brand Name: **NEO-SYNALAR**
- **Manufacturer:** Syntex
- **Use:** Skin infection, inflammation
- **Dosage Form:** Cream
- **Administration:** Topical
- **Ingredients:** Neomycin sulfate 0.5% (antibacterial); fluocinolone acetonide 0.025% (corticosteroid).

NEO-SYNALAR is an antibiotic-corticosteroid combination used to treat skin disorders that involve infection. The effectiveness of topical antibiotics, such as neomycin, is highly questionable. The use of corticosteroids for the treatment of skin infections may be dangerous because they can either mask the evidence of infection or cause the spreading of infections. Neomycin commonly causes skin rashes and can sensitize people to other more important antibiotics. Combination drugs like Neo-Synalar should never be used.

Also see Part II: Drugs Applied Directly to Skin, Eye or Ear

- **Brand Name: NICO-METRAZOL**
- **Manufacturer:** Knoll
- **Use:** Central nervous system stimulation
- **Dosage Form:** Tablet / Elixir
- **Administration:** Oral / Oral
- **Ingredients:** Pentylenetetrazol (stimulant/analeptic), nicotinic acid (vitamin); alcohol 15% (in elixir).

NICO-METRAZOL is a combination of a central nervous system (CNS) stimulant and a vitamin (with vasodilator properties) administered to enhance the mental and physical activity of elderly patients. Based on its purported cerebral (brain) vasodilation effects, it is promoted and used as a psychostimulant. Some doctors prescribe it for vertigo (dizziness) and a disease of the inner ear (Meniere's). Identical drugs include: Menic, Mentalert, Penalate, Scrip-Vasco, Senilex, Senilezol, Vazole.

- **Brand Name: NITRO-BID OINTMENT**
- **Manufacturer:** Marion
- **Use:** Heart pain (angina pectoris)
- **Dosage Form:** Ointment
- **Administration:** Topical
- **Ingredients:** Nitroglycerin 2% (coronary vasodilator).

NITRO-BID OINTMENT is promoted and prescribed for the prevention and treatment of chest pain associated with angina pectoris (transient pain due to coronary artery disease). Nitroglycerin is well absorbed through the skin. It affects the blood vessels within about 15 minutes, and lasts a variable length of time, often more than 1 hour.

Nitroglycerin ointment lacks evidence of effectiveness in treating acute attacks of angina whereas the sublingual tablet form is effective for this purpose. Although the FDA also considers nitroglycerin ointment to lack evidence of effectiveness in protecting against anginal attacks, one well-controlled study has found the ointment effective for this purpose (*Angiology* 27: 205-211, 1978). Identical drugs include: Nitrol.

Also see Part II: Drugs for Heart Pain

- Brand Name: **NITRO-BID PLATEAU CAPS**
- **Manufacturer:** Marion
- **Use:** Heart pain (angina pectoris)
- **Dosage Form:** Time-release capsule
- **Administration:** Oral
- **Ingredients:** Nitroglycerin 2.5, 6.5 or 9 mg (coronary vasodilator).

NITRO-BID, a time-release nitrate vasodilator, is promoted and prescribed for the prevention and control of transient pain due to coronary artery disease (angina pectoris). Nitroglycerin, when taken under the tongue, is the preferred drug for treatment of acute attacks of angina pectoris. However, despite heavy advertising claims to the contrary, there is no conclusive evidence that prolonged oral use of nitroglycerin or other oral nitrates in time-release preparations will diminish the severity and frequency of anginal attacks. Identical drugs include: Ang-O-Span, Dialex-2.5, Dialex-6.5, Gly-Trate Meta-Kaps, Nitrine-TDC, Nitro, Nitrobon-TR, Nitrocap-6.5, Nitrocap-T.D., Nitrocels Diacels, Nitrocot, Nitroglycerin, Nitrolin, Nitrospan, Nitrosule Pellsules, Nitro-T.D., Nitrotym, Nitrozem, Trates Granucaps, Vasoglyn Unicelles.

Also see Part II: Drugs for Heart Pain

- **Brand Name: NITROGLYN**
- **Manufacturer:** Key
- **Use:** Heart pain (angina pectoris)
- **Dosage Form:** Time-release tablets
- **Administration:** Oral
- **Ingredients:** Nitroglycerin 1.3, 2.6 or 6.5 mg (coronary vasodilator).

NITROGLYN is promoted and prescribed for the management, prevention or treatment of angina (pain due to coronary artery disease). As with all of the other oral (as opposed to sublingual, or under the tongue) nitrate vasodilators, there is no satisfactory evidence that Nitroglyn can prevent the onset of angina pectoris or diminish the frequency and/or severity of the attacks.

There is considerable controversy concerning the therapeutic value of these oral nitrate agents. None of the oral nitrate coronary vasodilator agents has been rated effective for the long-term treatment of angina pectoris. Identical drugs include: Nitro-Lor, Nitrong, Nitrovas.

Also see Part II: Drugs for Heart Pain

- **Brand Name: NUMORPHAN RECTAL SUPPOSITORIES**
- **Manufacturer:** Endo
- **Use:** Pain relief
- **Dosage Form:** Suppository
- **Administration:** Rectal
- **Ingredients:** Oxymorphone 5 mg (narcotic analgesic).

NUMORPHAN RECTAL SUPPOSITORIES are indicated for the relief of moderate to severe pain. Although the FDA has rated the intravenous form of oxymorphone (a derivative of morphine) "effective" for a wide variety of conditions associated with pain, the rectal suppository lacks sufficient evidence of efficacy and is, therefore, not recommended.

- **Brand Name: NYSTAFORM-HC**
- **Manufacturer:** Dome
- **Use:** Skin disorders
- **Dosage Form:** Ointment
- **Administration:** Topical
- **Ingredients:** Iodochlorhydroxyquin 1% (antibacterial); hydrocortisone 1% (corticosteroid); nystatin 100,000 u per gm (antifungal).

NYSTAFORM-HC is a fixed-combination product which was developed for the treatment of skin disorders involving fungal (yeast) infection, bacterial infections and inflammation. If a fungal infection is found to be present, nystatin may be useful as an antifungal agent, but it should be administered separately and not as part of a "shotgun" regimen. The use of corticosteroids for the treatment of skin infections may be dangerous because they can either mask the evidence of infection or cause the spreading of infections.

If hydrocortisone is needed for skin conditions, it should almost always be given alone. If a serious skin infection is present, it should be treated with the appropriate oral antibiotic, following a culture.

Also see Part II: Drugs Applied Directly to Skin, Eye or Ear

- **Brand Name: OMNI-TUSS**
- **Manufacturer:** Pennwalt
- **Use:** Cough and cold
- **Dosage Form:** Syrup
- **Administration:** Oral
- **Ingredients:** Codeine phosphate 10 mg (antitussive); phenyltoloxamine resin 5 mg, chlorpheniramine maleate 3 mg (antihistamines); ephedrine 25 mg (sympathomimetic); guaiacol carbonate 20 mg (expectorant) per 5 ml.

OMNI-TUSS is a polypharmaceutical mix used to treat cough in conditions such as common cold, acute bronchitis, allergic asthma and other respiratory disorders. Of the five separate ingredients contained in Omni-Tuss, only one, codeine, is a proven cough suppressant. The others include two antihistamines, a bronchodilator and an expectorant. The National Academy of Sciences-National Research Council rated this fixed-combination product ineffective for its labeled indications. Cough mixtures that contain antihistamines may thicken mucus and phlegm and thus interfere with a productive cough; moreover, antihistamines have no proven value in treating coughs or colds. The irrationality of this formulation is clearly demonstrated by the fact that two antihistamines are included together along with guaiacol carbonate, an expectorant, which is supposed to loosen secretions. Ephedrine can cause or aggravate high blood pressure and commonly loses it effectiveness when used regularly. Phenyltoloxamine and chlorpheniramine can cause drowsiness, loss of coordination, mental inattention and dizziness. Codeine often causes drowsiness and constipation and is psychologically and physically addicting when taken regularly.

Also see Part II: Drugs for Cough, Cold and Allergy

- **Brand Name: OPHTHOCORT**
- **Manufacturer:** Parke-Davis
- **Use:** Eye infection, inflammation
- **Dosage Form:** Ointment
- **Administration:** Eye
- **Ingredients:** Chloramphenicol 1%, polymyxin B sulfate 5000 u (antibacterials); hydrocortisone acetate .5% (corticosteroid) per gram.

OPHTHOCORT is promoted and used to treat various infections and inflammatory conditions of the eye and eyelid. This drug is certainly not appropriate for the treatment of these disorders. The use of a combined antibacterial/corticosteroid regimen may even worsen some eye infections (*AMA Drug Evaluations,* third edition, pg. 978). Moreover, corticosteroids lower resistance to infection and, by reducing inflammation, can mask the symptoms of serious eye disease.

WARNING: Chloramphenicol can cause serious and fatal blood disorders. Ophthocort should never be used and chloramphenicol alone should be limited to serious infections that do not respond to other antibacterial agents.

Also see Part II: Drugs Applied Directly to Skin, Eye or Ear

- **Brand Name:** ORENZYME
- **Manufacturer:** Merrell-National
- **Use:** Inflammation and edema
- **Dosage Form:** Enteric coated tablet
- **Administration:** Oral
- **Ingredients:** Trypsin, chymotrypsin (proteolytic enzymes).

ORENZYME has been found by the FDA to be lacking substantial evidence of efficacy for all of its labeled uses. These include relief of symptoms associated with episiotomy (incision made during childbirth to assist in delivery) and adjunctive therapy for inflammation and tissue swelling resulting from serious accidental or surgical injury.

Orenzyme is a fixed-combination comprised of two protein-digesting enzymes normally produced by the pancreas. Even the manufacturers concede that "the mode of action of Orenzyme has not been established."

- **Brand Name:** ORNADE SPANSULES
- **Manufacturer:** Smith Kline & French
- **Use:** Cough and cold
- **Dosage Form:** Time-release capsule
- **Administration:** Oral
- **Ingredients:** Isopropamide 2.5 mg (anticholinergic); chlorpheniramine maleate 8 mg (antihistamine); phenylpropanolamine hydrochloride 50 mg (sympathomimetic).

ORNADE is promoted to relieve upper respiratory tract congestion and hypersecretion associated with various allergic conditions and the common cold. Doctors prescribe it to combat sneezing, runny nose and other symptoms of nasal congestion. This fixed-combination product exemplifies the "shotgun" approach to treating cold symptoms. Sufficient clinical evidence of efficacy is lacking for the mixture.

Ornade is composed of an anticholinergic drug, an antihistamine and a sympathomimetic component. Because of its variable absorption and uneven course of action, the long-lasting capsule form is unacceptable. For congestion due to allergy, generic chlorpheniramine maleate alone is recommended. Isopropamide often causes blurring of vision, dryness of the mouth and throat, constipation and hesitancy of urination. Phenylpropanolamine can cause or aggravate high blood pressure and commonly loses its effectiveness when used regularly. Chlorpheniramine can cause drowsiness, loss of coordination, mental inattention and dizziness. Identical drugs include: Allernade (Improved) Capsules, Capade Capsules, Coryztime Improved Capsules, Decongestcaps, Vernate II Capsules.

Also see Part II: Drugs for Cough, Cold and Allergy

- **Brand Name: ORTHOXINE HYDROCHLORIDE**
- **Manufacturer:** Upjohn
- **Use:** Allergy and asthma
- **Dosage Form:** Tablet /Syrup
- **Administration:** Oral / Oral
- **Ingredients:** Methoxyphenamine hydrochloride (antihistamine).

ORTHOXINE HYDROCHLORIDE is a single-entity drug used to relieve the symptoms of various allergic conditions, including nasal mucosal, gastrointestinal and bronchial asthma. The FDA has reclassified this drug as lacking substantial evidence of effectiveness for its labeled indications and has taken the first step toward removing it from the market. Patients with allergy symptoms other than asthma would do best with an effective single-entity antihistamine, such as chlorpheniramine—but not in a long-acting form. Methoxyphenamine can cause drowsiness, loss of coordination, mental inattention and dizziness.

Also see Part II: Drugs for Cough, Cold and Allergy

- **Brand Name: OTOBIOTIC**
- **Manufacturer:** Schering
- **Use:** Ear infection
- **Dosage Form:** Solution
- **Administration:** Ear
- **Ingredients:** Neomycin sulfate 5 mg (antibacterial); sodium propionate 50 mg (antifungal) per ml.

OTOBIOTIC is used for the topical treatment of superficial bacterial infections of the external ear canal caused by susceptible organisms. Neomycin can produce skin sensitivity reactions as well as other toxic reactions when applied in the ear. Topical antibiotics of unproven effectiveness and questionable safety, such as neomycin, are not recommended in any instances.

Also see Part II: Drugs Applied Directly to Skin, Eye or Ear

- **Brand Name: OTOCORT**
- **Manufacturer:** Lemmon
- **Use:** Ear infection
- **Dosage Form:** Solution
- **Administration:** Ear
- **Ingredients:** Neomycin sulfate 5 mg, polymyxin B sulfate 2000 u (antibacterials); hydrocortisone 0.1% (corticosteroid); antipyrine 5%, dibucaine hydrochloride 0.25% (anesthetics) per ml.

OTOCORT is a fixed-combination drug product used to treat external ear infections and the associated pain and itching. It is composed of two antibacterials, a corticosteroid and two local anesthetics. Local anesthetics, such as dibucaine and antipyrine, are of questionable efficacy in ear solutions and may have adverse effects, such as sensitization (promoting allergy).

The use of topical antibiotics for wounds and infections is at best debatable, and furthermore, neomycin commonly causes skin rashes and can sensitize people to other, more important antibiotics. The use of corticosteroids for the treatment of skin infections may be dangerous because they can either mask the evidence of infection or cause the spreading of infections. Identical drugs include: My-Cort Otic, Otoreid-HC.

Also see Part II: Drugs Applied Directly to Skin, Eye or Ear

- **Brand Name: OXAINE M**
- **Manufacturer:** Wyeth
- **Use:** Stomach disorders and indigestion (heartburn)
- **Dosage Form:** Suspension
- **Administration:** Oral
- **Ingredients:** Oxethazaine 10 mg (local anesthetic); alumina gel (antacid).

OXAINE M combines an antacid with a potent topical local anesthetic (oxethazaine). It is used to relieve the pain associated with stomach ulcer and heartburn (esophagus inflammation). While this preparation may relieve symptoms of stomach and esophageal disorders, clinical studies do not indicate Oxaine M is any more effective than antacid therapy alone. Because oxethazaine has not been found to contribute to the effectiveness of the alumina gel antacid component and may also produce irritation, it is better (and less expensive) to use an antacid that doesn't include a local anesthetic.

The FDA has classified this product as ineffective and has initiated the process of withdrawing it from the market.

- **Brand Name: OXSORALEN**
- **Manufacturer:** Elder
- **Use:** Pigmentation disorders
- **Dosage Form:** Capsule
- **Administration:** Oral
- **Ingredients:** Methoxsalen 10 mg (pigmenting agent).

OXSORALEN is used to repigment those areas of skin which are completely lacking in natural pigment (melanin) due to a skin disease, vitiligo. However, Oxsoralen has been classified by the FDA as lacking substantial evidence of effectiveness.*

This drug is always used in combination with exposure to ultraviolet light. A recent study showed that patients receiving Oxsoralen therapy for psoriasis have a 2.5 times greater risk of getting skin cancer *(New Eng J Med,* 300: 809-13, 1979).

*Oxsoralen in lotion form is considered effective.

- **Brand Name: PAPASE**
- **Manufacturer:** Warner-Chilcott
- **Use:** Enzyme
- **Dosage Form:** Tablet
- **Administration:** Buccal
- **Ingredients:** Vegetable pepsin (proteolytic enzyme).

PAPASE is an extract of protein-degrading enzymes used to relieve the symptoms related to episiotomy (incision during childbirth to assist in delivery). The FDA has classified this product as lacking substantial evidence of effectiveness for its labeled indications and has begun the procedure to withdraw approval of its marketing.

- **Brand Name: PAPAVATRAL LA W/PHENOBARBITAL.**
- **Manufacturer:** Kenwood
- **Use:** Heart pain (angina pectoris)
- **Dosage Form:** Time-release capsule
- **Administration:** Oral
- **Ingredients:** Ethaverine hydrochloride 30 mg (vasodilator); pentaerythritol tetranitrate 50 mg (coronary vasodilator); phenobarbital 45 mg (sedative).

PAPAVATRAL LA W/PHENOBARBITAL is a fixed-combination drug product promoted and prescribed for the prevention, control and treatment of the pain of coronary artery disease (angina pectoris). It is prescribed when the physician believes that anxiety or emotional disturbance may be important factors in the clinical situation, hence the inclusion of a sedative (phenobarbital) in the drug mixture. In addition to phenobarbital, Papavatral LA is composed of two agents which act to dilate blood vessels. Ethaverine, a derivative of papaverine, is a non-specific vasodilator; pentaerythritol tetranitrate is claimed by the drug companies to be a particularly effective vasodilator at the level of the coronary (heart) arteries. However, there is no satisfactory clinical evidence that either of these drugs, taken alone or in combination, is of any therapeutic value in long-term prevention or management of heart pain.

   For relief of acute anginal attacks, or to decrease the likelihood of an attack during a period of strenuous physical activity, one may take nitroglycerin under the tongue. Sedatives, such as phenobarbital, may help some people with angina pectoris; however, if they are truly needed, they should be administered separately at the appropriate dose. At this point, there is no sound clinical evidence that the daily use of sedatives contributes positively to treating angina. Moreover, the amount of phenobarbital included in this combination (45 mg) could make one too drowsy to be able to function well. When taken regularly, phenobarbital can lead to psychological and physical addiction. There is strong evidence that ethaverine causes liver damage in many people *(New Eng J Med* 281: 1333-35 and 1364-65, 1969).

Also see Part II: Drugs for Heart Pain

- Brand Name: **PAPAVERINE**
- **Manufacturer:** generic
- **Use:** Blood vessel disease (head and limbs)
- **Dosage Form:** Time-release capsule /Tablet /Solution
- **Administration:** Oral / Oral / Injection
- **Ingredients:** Papaverine hydrochloride (vasodilator).

PAPAVERINE is the prototype of the vasodilators and is available generically in a number of dosage forms from a variety of drug manufacturing firms. It is promoted for vascular (blood vessel) diseases associated with insufficient blood flow resulting from either blocked arteries or blood vessel spasm (constriction). Papaverine products are usually administered to elderly patients for peripheral (arms and legs) and cerebral (brain) vascular diseases. These drugs are heralded by the manufacturers as having specific efficacy in preserving blood circulation to the brain, in preventing vessel spasm that might result in brain damage and in relieving and reducing symptoms after cerebral damage. However, there is no convincing evidence that papaverine or related products have any therapeutic value in these conditions. There is strong evidence that papaverine can cause liver damage in many people (*New Eng J Med* 281: 1333-35 and 1364-65, 1969). Identical drugs include: P-200, V-Pav.

Also see Part II: Drugs for Circulatory Disorders of Head and Limbs

- **Brand Name: PARAFON FORTE**
- **Manufacturer:** McNeil
- **Use:** Pain relief (musculoskeletal conditions)
- **Dosage Form:** Tablet
- **Administration:** Oral
- **Ingredients:** Chlorzoxazone 250 mg (muscle relaxant); acetaminophen 300 mg (analgesic).

PARAFON FORTE is used in addition to rest and physical therapy for relief of discomfort from acute, painful, musculoskeletal conditions such as sprain and back pain. How this drug works has not been clearly identified and the principal ingredient, chlorzoxazone, has not been shown to be a "muscle relaxant." Any effect is probably due to the acetaminophen (as in Tylenol) content. The *AMA Drug Evaluations* (second edition, p. 274) states, "the rationale for use of the preparation is highly questionable." Identical drugs include: Chlorofon-F, Chlorzone Forte, Chlorzoxazone w/APAP, Lobac, Parachlor, Tuzon.

- **Brand Name: PARNATE**
- **Manufacturer:** Smith Kline & French
- **Use:** Anti-depressant
- **Dosage Form:** Tablet
- **Administration:** Oral
- **Ingredients:** Tranylcypromine sulfate 10 mg (monoamine oxidase inhibitor).

PARNATE is used to relieve the symptoms of severe depression in hospitalized or closely supervised patients who have not responded to other anti-depressant therapy. This single-entity drug, known as a monoamine oxidase inhibitor, lacks evidence of effectiveness. As the FDA admits, most people with drug-responsive depression will improve when given other medicines (the "tricyclic antidepressants") which are less dangerous.

WARNING: Fatal reactions to this drug (hypertensive crises) can occur when it is used with drugs such as amphetamines or with cheese, beer, wine and other foods.

- **Brand Name: PATHIBAMATE**
- **Manufacturer:** Lederle
- **Use:** Digestive disorders
- **Dosage Form:** Tablet
- **Administration:** Oral
- **Ingredients:** Tridihexethyl chloride 25 mg (antispasmodic/anti-secretory); meprobamate 200 or 400 mg (sedative).

PATHIBAMATE, in both dosage forms, is used as adjunctive therapy in stomach ulcer and irritable bowel syndrome, especially when accompanied by anxiety or tension. However, there is insufficient clinical evidence to support these efficacy claims. Pathibamate has not proven effective in relieving ulcer pain or hastening the healing of ulcers. If anxiety and stress are in fact sources of gastrointestinal problems, and if a sedative drug or tranquilizer is appropriate, it is preferable to use the safest drug at the lowest effective dose. Meprobamate is not the best drug. Tridihexethyl chloride often causes blurring of vision, dryness of the mouth and throat, constipation and hesitancy of urination. Identical drugs include: Milpath, Spasmate, Spenpath, Tri-Hexabamate, Tridihexethyl Chloride w/Meprobamate.

WARNING: The use of minor tranquilizers such as meprobamate (Miltown), chlordiazepoxide (Librium), diazepam (Valium) or similar drugs during pregnancy should be avoided because of increased risk of damage to the developing fetus. One must consider the possibility of pregnancy when beginning minor tranquilizer therapy. In the case of combination drugs such as Pathibamate, use at any time is unwarranted.

Also see Part II: Drugs for Digestive Disorders

- **Brand Name:** **PATHILON W/PHENOBARBITAL**
- **Manufacturer:** Lederle
- **Use:** Digestive disorders
- **Dosage Form:** Tablet
- **Administration:** Oral
- **Ingredients:** Tridihexethyl chloride 25 mg (antispasmodic/antisecretory); phenobarbital 15 mg (sedative).

PATHILON W/PHENOBARBITAL

is used as an adjunct in the treatment of stomach ulcer, irritable bowel syndrome and other bowel disorders, especially when accompanied by anxiety or tension. However, this mixture has never demonstrated adequate evidence of effectiveness. There is no evidence at this time that this combination relieves ulcer pain or hastens healing, according to the *AMA Drug Evaluations* (third edition, pg. 1054). In addition, sedatives like phenobarbital, when taken regularly, can lead to psychological and physical addiction. Tridihexethyl chloride often causes blurring of vision, dryness of the mouth and throat, constipation and hesitancy of urination.

Also see Part II: Drugs for Digestive Disorders

- **Brand Name:** **PATHILON SEQUELS**
- **Manufacturer:** Lederle
- **Use:** Digestive disorders
- **Dosage Form:** Time-release capsule
- **Administration:** Oral
- **Ingredients:** Tridihexethyl chloride 75 mg (antispasmodic/antisecretory).

PATHILON SEQUELS is a time-release form of

tridihexethyl chloride, an antispasmodic/antisecretory drug. It is used to treat stomach ulcer, irritable bowel syndrome and other bowel disturbances. There is insufficient evidence that this time-release form contributes any added clinical benefit and also scant clinical evidence that tridihexethyl chloride relieves ulcer pain or speeds healing. Moreover, the effect of drugs such as tridihexethyl chloride on lessening intestinal over-activity, claimed to be one of the principal beneficial drug actions, is usually minimal.[1] Tridihexethyl chloride often causes blurring of vision, dryness of the mouth and throat, constipation and hesitancy of urination.

[1]Melmon KL, Morrelli HF. *Clinical Pharmacology,* 2nd ed., 435, 1972.

Also see Part II: Drugs for Digestive Disorders

- Brand Name: **PAVABID HP**
- **Manufacturer:** Marion
- **Use:** Blood vessel disease (head and limbs)
- **Dosage Form:** Tablet
- **Administration:** Oral
- **Ingredients:** Papaverine hydrochloride 300 mg (vasodilator).

PAVABID HP is similar to Pavabid Plateau except it comes in tablet form instead of capsule and it contains twice the dosage of papaverine. Pavabid HP is used to treat disorders due to insufficient blood flow primarily to the head and limbs and less frequently to the heart.

There is currently no evidence that papaverines work for any of their recommended uses and there is strong evidence that papaverines cause liver damage in many people (*New Eng J Med* 281:1333-35 and 1364-65, 1969). Identical drugs include: Pavagen-300.

See similar drug PAPAVERINE, pg. 143

Also see Part II: Drugs for Circulatory Disorders of Head and Limbs

- **Brand Name: PAVABID PLATEAU**
- **Manufacturer:** Marion
- **Use:** Blood vessel disease (head and limbs)
- **Dosage Form:** Time-release capsule
- **Administration:** Oral
- **Ingredients:** Papaverine hydrochloride 150 mg (vasodilator).

PAVABID PLATEAU is prescribed to obtain three principal actions: (1) general blood vessel dilation, (2) brain blood vessel dilation, (3) coronary artery dilation. Manufacturers claim that Pavabid and related drug products are effective for nearly any condition known to involve impaired circulation, such as senility, leg cramping and light-headedness in older patients. Pavabid is the largest-selling papaverine drug product. However, there is no satisfactory evidence that Pavabid and related drug products have any therapeutic value. There is strong evidence that these drugs cause liver damage in many people (*New Eng J Med* 281: 1333-35 and 1364-65, 1969). Identical drugs include: Blupav, Cerebid-TD, Cerespan, Delapav, Dilart, Dipav, Kavrin, K-Pava, Lapav Graduals, Myobid, Orapav Timecelles, Papacon, Pap-Kaps-150 Meta-Kaps, Pavacap Unicelles, Pavacels, Pavacen Cenules, Pavacot T.D., Pavacron, Pavadur, Pavadyl, Pavakey, Pava-Mead, Pava-Par, Pava-Rx, Pavased, Pavasule, Pavatran, Pava-2, Pavatym, Pava-Wol, Paverine Spancaps, Paverolan, Sustaverine, Tri-Pavasule, Vasal Granucaps, Vasocap-150, Vasospan.

Also see Part II: Drugs for Circulatory Disorders of Head and Limbs

- **Brand Name: PAVAKEY-300**
- **Manufacturer:** Key
- **Use:** Blood vessel disease (head and limbs)
- **Dosage Form:** Time-release capsule
- **Administration:** Oral
- **Ingredients:** Papaverine hydrochloride 300 mg (vasodilator).

PAVAKEY-300, which contains twice the usual amount of papaverine in a so-called time-release formulation, is equally as ineffective as other papaverine drugs containing 150 mg of the ingredient. Also, there is strong evidence that papaverine causes liver damage in many people (*New Eng J Med* 281: 1333-35 and 1364-65, 1969). Identical drugs include: Cerebid-300 TD, Dilart-

300, Pavacels-300, Pavadyl-300, Pavasule Forte, Pavatran-300, PT-300, Tri-Pavasule 300, Vasocap-300.

See similar drugs PAVABID PLATEAU, pg. 148, and PAPAVERINE, pg. 143

Also see Part II: Drugs for Circulatory Disorders of Head and Limbs

- Brand Name: **PAVERIL PHOSPHATE**
- **Manufacturer:** Lilly
- **Use:** Heart pain (angina pectoris)
- **Dosage Form:** Tablet
- **Administration:** Oral
- **Ingredients:** Dioxyline phosphate 100 or 200 mg (vasodilator).

PAVERIL PHOSPHATE is used to treat angina pectoris (transient chest pain due to coronary artery disease) and spasm of blood vessels in arms, legs or lungs. There is no conclusive evidence to support claims of efficacy in the case of angina pectoris. Dioxyline phosphate nonspecifically relaxes vascular (blood vessel) smooth muscle. Yet it is not potent when given orally, and its efficacy in the treatment of peripheral (arms and legs) vascular disorders is highly dubious.

Also see Part II: Drugs for Heart Pain
Drugs for Circulatory Disorders of Head and Limbs

- Brand Name: **PBZ W/EPHEDRINE**
- **Manufacturer:** Geigy
- **Use:** Allergy and congestion
- **Dosage Form:** Tablet
- **Administration:** Oral
- **Ingredients:** Tripelennamine hydrochloride 25 mg (antihistamine); ephedrine sulfate 12 mg (sympathomimetic).

PBZ W/EPHEDRINE is a combination product promoted and used for the treatment of hay fever. Tripelennamine, an antihistamine, is considered effective for treating allergy symptoms in doses of 25-50 mg. Ephedrine, however, has not been conclusively shown to confer significant therapeutic value to patients suffering from hay fever and allergic conditions.

Ephedrine can cause or aggravate high blood pressure and commonly loses its effectiveness when used regularly. Tripelennamine can cause drowsiness, loss of coordination, mental inattention and dizziness.

Also see Part II: Drugs for Cough, Cold and Allergy

- Brand Name: **PBZ EXPECTORANT W/EPHEDRINE**
- **Manufacturer:** Geigy
- **Use:** Cough and asthma
- **Dosage Form:** Syrup
- **Administration:** Oral
- **Ingredients:** Tripelennamine citrate 37.5 mg (antihistamine); ephedrine sulfate 12.5 mg (sympathomimetic); ammonium chloride 100 mg (expectorant) per 5 ml.

PBZ EXPECTORANT W/EPHEDRINE is marketed to relieve persistent, dry cough accompanying colds and allergic respiratory disorders. It is also used to treat some cases of asthma. However, its formulation lacks a genuine cough-suppressing agent, such as dextromethorphan, and may only be considered inappropriate for its labeled indications. It has been rated ineffective by a National Academy of Sciences-National Research Council scientific panel.

Although ephedrine sulfate is sometimes used to treat asthma, it should be taken separately for this medical problem. Moreover, the antihistamine, tripelennamine, has not shown substantial evidence of efficacy in suppressing cough. All drugs are potentially unsafe and only if the potential benefit of a medicine outweighs those risks should one use it. PBZ Expectorant with Ephedrine is of no proven benefit to a patient with a cough, so one can justify neither the risks of side effects nor the costs.

Ephedrine can cause or aggravate high blood pressure and commonly loses its effectiveness when used regularly. Tripelennamine can cause drowsiness, loss of coordination, mental inattention and dizziness. Ammonium chloride can be harmful to patients with improperly functioning lungs, liver, or kidneys.

Also see Part II: Drugs for Cough, Cold and Allergy

- **Brand Name:** PBZ EXPECTORANT W/EPHEDRINE AND CODEINE
- **Manufacturer:** Geigy
- **Use:** Cough and cold
- **Dosage Form:** Syrup
- **Administration:** Oral
- **Ingredients:** Codeine phosphate 8 mg (antitussive/narcotic); tripelennamine citrate 30 mg (antihistamine); ephedrine sulfate 10 mg (sympathomimetic); ammonium chloride 80 mg (expectorant).

PBZ EXPECTORANT W/EPHEDRINE AND CODEINE is

promoted and used for the control of cough. It contains the narcotic codeine, which is an effective cough suppressant (although the use of the effective non-narcotic dextromethorphan is preferable). However, the inclusion of tripelennamine citrate, an antihistamine, and ephedrine sulfate, a bronchodilator, is highly questionable. This product was designated as ineffective as a fixed-combination by a National Academy of Sciences-National Research Council scientific panel. Use of this mixed-bag product is an example of sloppy medical practice, since it contains unnecessary and ineffective drug components and exposes the patient to unnecessary risks. Ephedrine can cause or aggravate high blood pressure and commonly loses its effectiveness when used regularly. Tripelennamine can cause drowsiness, loss of coordination, mental inattention and dizziness. Codeine often causes drowsiness and constipation and is psychologically and physically addicting when taken regularly. Ammonium chloride can be harmful to people with improperly functioning lungs, liver or kidneys.

Also see Part II: Drugs for Cough, Cold and Allergy

- **Brand Name: PBZ LONTABS AND PBZ-SR**
- **Manufacturer:** Geigy
- **Use:** Cold and allergy
- **Dosage Form:** Time-release tablet
- **Administration:** Oral
- **Ingredients:** Tripelennamine hydrochloride 50 or 100 mg (antihistamine).

PBZ LONTABS AND PBZ-SR are used to

treat hay fever and a wide variety of allergic conditions. In general, tripelennamine is an effective antihistamine for allergy symptoms, but is expensive to buy in these forms. Instead, it should be purchased by its generic name, tripelennamine. The time-release form is not recommended because its alleged longer action is uneven, its additional cost is unnecessary, and there is insufficient evidence that it confers significant therapeutic benefit to the patient. Tripelennamine can cause drowsiness, loss of coordination, mental inattention and dizziness.

Also see Part II: Drugs for Cough, Cold and Allergy

- **Brand Name: PENTRITOL**
- **Manufacturer:** Armour
- **Use:** Heart pain (angina pectoris)
- **Dosage Form:** Time-release capsule
- **Administration:** Oral
- **Ingredients:** Pentaerythritol tetranitrate 30 or 60 mg (coronary vasodilator).

PENTRITOL is a time-release form of the coronary vaso-

dilator pentaerythritol tetranitrate, used for the prevention and/or treatment of transient chest pain (angina pectoris) due to coronary artery disease. Evidence from careful clinical studies that pentaerythritol tetranitrate and similar oral nitrate vasodilators are successful in preventing angina has not been forthcoming. Adequate evidence is lacking to support the general efficacy claims made by the manufacturers of Pentritol and similar drugs.

Also see Part II: Drugs for Heart Pain

- **Brand Name: PENTRYATE STRONGER**
- **Manufacturer:** Fellows
- **Use:** Heart pain (angina pectoris)
- **Dosage Form:** Time-release capsule
- **Administration:** Oral
- **Ingredients:** Pentaerythritol tetranitrate 80 mg (coronary vasodilator).

PENTRYATE STRONGER is a time-release form of the coronary vasodilator pentaerythritol tetranitrate, used for the prevention and/or treatment of transient chest pain (angina pectoris) due to coronary artery disease. Evidence from careful clinical studies that pentaerythritol tetranitrate and similar oral nitrate vasodilators are successful in preventing angina has not been forthcoming. Adequate evidence is lacking to support the general efficacy claims made by the manufacturers of Pentryate and similar drugs. Identical drugs include: Desatrate 80, Kaytrate-80, Naptrate Spancap, Neo-Corovas-80 Tymcaps, Pentaerythritol Tetranitrate, Pentetra-80 TDC, Pentraspan-80, Pentryate-80, P.E.T.N., Vaso-80 Unicelles.

Also see Part II: Drugs for Heart Pain

- **Brand Name: PERITRATE**
- **Manufacturer:** Parke-Davis
- **Use:** Heart pain (angina pectoris)
- **Dosage Form:** Time-release tablet / Tablet
- **Administration:** Oral / Oral
- **Ingredients:** Pentaerythritol tetranitrate 10, 20, 40 or 80 mg (coronary vasodilator).

PERITRATE has never been rated effective as a long-term therapy in the management of angina pectoris (transient pain due to coronary artery disease). Evidence that it is useful in preventing and diminishing the frequency and severity of anginal episodes remains insufficient. Identical drugs include: Angijen, Angijen-20, Angitrate #10, Angitrate #20, Naptrate, Pentaerythritol Tetranitrate, Pentylan, Perihab, P.E.T.N., Rate-10, Rate-20, Reithritol.

Also see Part II: Drugs for Heart Pain

- **Brand Name: PERITRATE W/PHENOBARBITAL**
- **Manufacturer:** Parke-Davis
- **Use:** Heart pain (angina pectoris)
- **Dosage Form:** Tablet /Time-release tablet
- **Administration:** Oral / Oral
- **Ingredients:** Pentaerythritol tetranitrate 10 or 20 mg (coronary vasodilator); phenobarbital 15 mg (sedative).

PERITRATE W/PHENOBARBITAL

is sold for the prevention, control and treatment of the pain of coronary artery disease (angina pectoris). The manufacturer recommends it especially when the physican believes anxiety or emotional disturbances may be important factors in causing angina. Peritrate, in all of its dosage forms, has been rated by the FDA as lacking substantial evidence of efficacy for its labeled uses. Sedatives such as phenobarbital may help some people with angina pectoris by reducing the anxiety and tension that might precipitate anginal attacks. If they are needed, however, they should be administered separately, in doses adjusted to each person's specific needs. The chronic use of phenobarbital may produce both psychological and physical addiction. Its routine use by patients with angina is not recommended. Identical drugs include: Pentaerythritol Tetranitrate w/Phenobarbital.

Also see Part II: Drugs for Heart Pain

- **Brand Name: PERSANTINE**
- **Manufacturer:** Boehringer-Ingelheim
- **Use:** Heart pain (angina pectoris)
- **Dosage Form:** Tablet
- **Administration:** Oral
- **Ingredients:** Dipyridamole 25 mg (coronary vasodilator).

PERSANTINE

is promoted and commonly prescribed for "long-term therapy" of chronic angina pectoris (transient pain of coronary artery disease). However, manufacturer's claims that prolonged therapy may reduce the frequency or severity of anginal attacks, improve exercise tolerance, and reduce nitroglycerin requirement remain unproven. Persantine is certainly not effective in treating acute angina and it has never been rated effective for any indication.

According to the *AMA Drug Evaluations* (second edition, pg. 21), Persantine "increases the coronary blood flow in animals, but is of no value in treating an acute attack of angina pectoris. The evidence that its long-term administration will be beneficial in patients with angina pectoris is not convincing." That judgment, made in 1973, has not been refuted. Persantine remains a very expensive drug of unproven effectiveness.

At present there are some medical scientists who believe that Persantine may be beneficial for preventing heart attack and stroke in the patient with the usual kind of angina.[1] It has been shown in one study that aspirin and dipyridamole inhibit the blood clotting process by keeping platelets (components of blood that help to form clots during normal repair) from sticking together in the test tube. These drugs are currently being tested to see if together they can prevent problems like heart attacks and strokes, which are thought to be caused—at least in part—by abnormal blood clotting.

Although studies of the anti-clotting action of Persantine are underway and one study[2] has demonstrated a decreased rate of heart attacks among anginal patients, this drug has not been approved by the FDA as an effective medication for preventing heart attacks. Identical drugs include: Dipyridamole.

[1] *Medical World News* 201(16):42-48, 1979.
[2] *New Eng J Med,* 1978.

Also see Part II: Drugs for Heart Pain

- Brand Name: **PHENERGAN EXPECTORANT W/CODEINE**
- **Manufacturer:** Wyeth
- **Use:** Cough, cold, allergy
- **Dosage Form:** Syrup
- **Administration:** Oral
- **Ingredients:** Codeine phosphate 10 mg (antitussive/narcotic); promethazine hydrochloride 5 mg (antihistamine/sedative); ipecac fluid extract .1 ml, potassium guaiacolsulfonate 44 mg, citric acid 60 mg, sodium citrate 197 mg (expectorants) per 5 ml; alcohol 7%.

PHENERGAN EXPECTORANT W/CODEINE is used in the treatment of cough. This

particular formulation differs from Phenergan Expectorant Plain in that it contains the effective cough-suppressing agent codeine phosphate. Promethazine, an antihistamine with powerful sedative-antinausea properties, is useful for treating nausea and allergic conditions. However, all of the other ingredients in this combination product lack evidence of therapeutic efficacy. Multi-drug preparations such as this and all of the Phenergan line can only be condemned as "shotgun" remedies and should not be used. Most coughs that should be treated can be satisfactorily quieted by dextromethorphan, a non-narcotic antitussive agent that is available without a prescription.

The National Academy of Sciences-National Research Council has rated this product ineffective as a fixed-combination. Ipecac fluid extract does not belong in a cough and cold preparation. Codeine often causes drowsiness and constipation and is psychologically and physically addicting when taken regularly. Promethazine can cause drowsiness, loss of coordination, mental inattention and dizziness. Identical drugs include: K-Phen Expectorant w/Codeine, Mallergan Expectorant w/Codeine, Pentazine Expectorant w/ Codeine, Promethazine HCl Expectorant w/Codeine, Promex w/ Codeine Expectorant, Prothazine w/Codeine Expectorant.

See SYNALGOS, pg. 174, for discussion of promethazine toxicity.

Also see Part II: Drugs for Cough, Cold and Allergy

- **Brand Name: PHENERGAN EXPECTORANT PEDIATRIC W/ DEXTROMETHORPHAN**

- **Manufacturer:** Wyeth
- **Use:** Cough, cold, allergy
- **Dosage Form:** Syrup
- **Administration:** Oral
- **Ingredients:** Dextromethorphan 7.5 mg (antitussive); promethazine hydrochloride 5 mg (antihistamine/sedative); ipecac fluid extract .1 ml, potassium guaiacolsulfonate 44 mg, citric acid 60 mg, sodium citrate 197 mg (expectorants) per 5 ml; alcohol 7%.

PHENERGAN EXPECTORANT PEDIATRIC W/DEXTROMETHORPHAN is similar to

Phenergan VC Expectorant with Codeine. With this product, Wyeth has merely substituted dextromethorphan, a non-narcotic cough-suppressing agent, for codeine. It has been promoted for children. Promethazine can cause drowsiness, loss of coordination, mental inattention and dizziness. Identical drugs include: Prothazine Pediatric Liquid.

See similar drug PHENERGAN VC EXPECTORANT WITH CODEINE, pg. 158

Also see Part II: Drugs for Cough, Cold and Allergy

- **Brand Name: PHENERGAN EXPECTORANT PLAIN**
- **Manufacturer:** Wyeth
- **Use:** Cough, cold, allergy
- **Dosage Form:** Syrup
- **Administration:** Oral
- **Ingredients:** Promethazine hydrochloride 5 mg (antihistamine/sedative); ipecac fluid extract .1 ml, potassum guaiacolsulfonate 44 mg, citric acid 60 mg, sodium citrate 197 mg (expectorants) per 5 ml; alcohol 7%.

PHENERGAN EXPECTORANT PLAIN is used most often to treat cough. The principal ingredi-

ent, promethazine, is an effective antihistamine with powerful sedative); ipecac fluid extract .1 ml, potassium guaiacolsulfonate 44 drugs is not recommended and has no proper role in treating coughs and viral colds. Phenergan is just a "shotgun" potpourri and, as a fixed-combination, it was rated ineffective by the National Academy of Sciences-National Research Council. Ipecac fluid extract has no place in a cough and cold medication. Promethazine can cause drowsiness, loss of coordination, mental inattention and dizziness. Identical drugs include: Mallergan Expectorant Plain, Pentazine Expectorant Plain, Promethazine HCl Expectorant Plain, Promex Expectorant, Prothazine Expectorant.

See SYNALGOS, pg. 174, for discussion of promethazine toxicity.

Also see Part II: Drugs for Cough, Cold and Allergy

- **Brand Name:** PHENERGAN VC EXPECTORANT W/ CODEINE
- **Manufacturer:** Wyeth
- **Use:** Cough and cold
- **Dosage Form:** Syrup
- **Administration:** Oral
- **Ingredients:** Codeine phosphate 10 mg (antitussive/narcotic); promethazine hydrochloride 5 mg (antihistamine/sedative); phenylephrine hydrochloride 5 mg (sympathomimetic); ipecac fluid extract .1 ml, potassium guaiacolsulfonate 44 mg, citric acid 60 mg, sodium citrate 197 mg (expectorants) per 5 ml; alcohol 7%.

PHENERGAN VC EXPECTORANT W/CODEINE

contains codeine phosphate, an agent used to suppress coughs, as well as phenylephrine hydrochloride and the standard five ingredients in Phenergan. Phenergan VC with Codeine has been cited as ineffective by a NAS-NRC scientific panel. Yet the FDA has allowed this and the other Phenergan products to remain on the market. Phenylephrine can cause or aggravate high blood pressure and commonly loses its effectiveness when used regularly while promethazine can cause drowsiness, loss of coordination, mental inattention and dizziness. Codeine often causes drowsiness and constipation and is psychologically and physically addicting when taken regularly. Identical drugs include: Mallergan-VC Expectorant w/Codeine, Pentazine VC Expectorant w/Codeine, Promethazine HCl VC Expectorant w/Codeine.

See similar drug PHENERGAN EXPECTORANT PLAIN, pg. 157

Also see Part II: Drugs for Cough, Cold and Allergy

- **Brand Name: PHENERGAN VC EXPECTORANT PLAIN**
- **Manufacturer:** Wyeth
- **Use:** Cough, cold, allergy
- **Dosage Form:** Syrup
- **Administration:** Oral
- **Ingredients:** Promethazine hydrochloride 5 mg (antihistamine/ sedative); phenylephrine hydrochloride 5 mg (sympathomimetic); ipecac fluid extract .1 ml, potassium guaiacolsulfonate 44 mg, citric acid 60 mg, sodium citrate 197 mg (expectorants), per 5 ml; alcohol 7%.

PHENERGAN VC EXPECTORANT PLAIN

PLAIN is composed of all the Phenergan Expectorant ingredients plus phenylephrine hydrochloride, a vasoconstrictor used for nasal decongestion. This product is promoted for all of the labeled indications of Phenergan Expectorant Plain, but is also intended to relieve nasal congestion and runny nose due to the common cold and allergies. Like all of the Phenergan products listed in this guide, the "VC" formulation is an irrational and potentially hazardous mixture. Ipecac fluid extract does not belong in a cough and cold medication. Phenergan VC Expectorant Plain was rated as ineffective by the NAS-NRC scientific panel. Relief from nasal congestion and related symptoms can be obtained by using generic phenylephrine hydrochloride nose drops. Phenylephrine can cause or aggravate high blood pressure and commonly loses its effectiveness when used regularly, while promethazine can cause drowsiness, loss of coordination, mental inattention and dizziness. Identical drugs include: Promethazine HCl VC Expectorant Plain.

See SYNALGOS, pg. 174, for discussion of promethazine toxicity.

Also see Part II: Drugs for Cough, Cold and Allergy

- **Brand Name: PHENOBARBITAL W/ ATROPINE**
- **Manufacturer:** generic
- **Use:** Digestive disorders
- **Dosage Form:** Tablet
- **Administration:** Oral
- **Ingredients:** Atropine sulfate 4 or 8 mg (antispasmodic/antisecretory); phenobarbital 15 or 30 mg (sedative).

PHENOBARBITAL W/ATROPINE

is a combination of an antispasmodic/antisecretory agent and a sedative. It is used by doctors to treat a variety of digestive disorders, including stomach ulcer and irritable bowel syndrome (a condition involving spasms of the large intestines often thought to be associated with nervous tension).

Phenobarbital with Atropine is one of many drug products listed in this guide that contains an antispasmodic/antisecretory agent in combination with a fixed amount of a sedative. The two drug components individually at the proper doses may be effective. However, there is insufficient evidence that the addition of sedatives to antispasmodic/antisecretory agents in fixed-ratios as in these products confers significant therapeutic benefit to the patient. When taken regularly, sedatives like phenobarbital can lead to psychological and physical addiction. Atropine often causes blurring of vision, dryness of the mouth and throat, constipation and hesitancy of urination. Identical drugs include: Phenobarbital and Belladonna.

Also see Part II: Drugs for Digestive Disorders

- **Brand Name: POTABA**
- **Manufacturer:** Glenwood
- **Use:** Skin and muscle disorders
- **Dosage Form:** Tablet /Capsule/ Powder
- **Administration:** Oral / Oral / Topical
- **Ingredients:** Potassium P-aminobenzoate (antifibrotic).

POTABA,

in its various dosage forms, is used to treat a number of skin and muscle diseases characterized by inappropriate inflammation and scar tissue formation (fibrosis).

In 1977, the FDA proposed to withdraw Potaba from the market, but Potaba continues to be sold as an antifibrotic drug.

- **Brand Name: PRISCOLINE**
- **Manufacturer:** Ciba
- **Use:** Blood vessel disease (head and limbs)
- **Dosage Form:** Tablet /Solution
- **Administration:** Oral/ Intravenous
- **Ingredients:** Tolazoline hydrochloride (vasodilator).

PRISCOLINE is used to treat peripheral blood vessel spasm associated with a broad spectrum of diseases, including claudications (cramping and weakness in the legs). However, there is a dearth of substantial evidence of Priscoline's clinical efficacy for its labeled uses. In a recent article published in the *New England Journal of Medicine,* Dr. J.D. Coffman reported that tolazoline "has not been of benefit in obstructive arterial diseases."[1] For the only problem where this drug has some potential use, Raynaud's syndrome (pallor of hands and feet induced by the cold), he reports that tolazoline is "occasionally useful" in combination with other agents. However, this particular use of Priscoline represents a tiny fraction of the total number of prescriptions written each year. Identical drugs include: Tolazoline, Vasodil.

[1] 300(13): 713-717, 1979.

Also see Part II: Drugs for Circulatory Disorders of Head and Limbs

- **Brand Name: PRISCOLINE LONTABS**
- **Manufacturer:** Ciba
- **Use:** Blood vessel disease (head and limbs)
- **Dosage Forms:** Time-release tablet
- **Administration:** Oral
- **Ingredients:** Tolazoline hydrochloride 80 mg (vasodilator).

PRISCOLINE LONTABS, like the other dosage forms of tolazoline, lack substantial evidence of clinical efficacy. A recent article on the status of the peripheral vasodilator drugs in obstructive vascular disease (the overwhelming usage) reveals little substantial evidence to support their use. They are not effective in the treatment of either intermittent claudication (cramp-like pain and weakness in legs) or ischemic symptoms at rest.[1]

[1] *N Eng J Med* 300(13): 713-717, 1979.

See similar drug PRISCOLINE, pg. 161

Also see Part II: Drugs for Circulatory Disorders of Head and Limbs

- **Brand Name: PRO-BANTHINE W/ DARTAL**
- **Manufacturer:** Searle
- **Use:** Digestive disorders
- **Dosage Form:** Tablet
- **Administration:** Oral
- **Ingredients:** Propantheline bromide 15 mg (antispasmodic/antisecretory); thiopropazate hydrochloride 5 mg (tranquilizer).

PRO-BANTHINE W/DARTAL is used as
back-up therapy in the treatment of stomach ulcer and other gastrointestinal disorders. The agent propantheline bromide supposedly acts to decrease the secretion of stomach acid and to slow the transport of food through the stomach and intestine. As a fixed-combination, this product has not demonstrated satisfactory evidence of clinical efficacy, according to the FDA. Propantheline often causes blurring of vision, dryness of the mouth and throat, constipation and hesitancy of urination.

Also see Part II: Drugs for Digestive Disorders

- **Brand Name: PRO-BANTHINE W/ PHENOBARBITAL**
- **Manufacturer:** Searle
- **Use:** Digestive disorders
- **Dosage Form:** Tablet
- **Administration:** Oral
- **Ingredients:** Propantheline bromide 15 mg (antispasmodic/antisecretory); phenobarbital 15 mg (sedative).

PRO-BANTHINE W/ PHENOBARBITAL is employed as adjunctive
therapy in the treatment of stomach ulcer and irritable bowel syndrome. In this product one finds the sedative phenobarbital combined with the antispasmodic/antisecretory agent propantheline. There is no satisfactory evidence that this mixture has any beneficial effect on ulcer patients beyond that afforded by an antacid or antispasmodic/antisecretory agent alone in proper dosage. In addition, when taken regularly, sedatives like phenobarbital can lead to psychological and physical addiction. Propantheline often causes blurring of vision, dryness of the mouth and throat, constipation and hesitancy of urination.

Also see Part II: Drugs for Digestive Disorders

- **Brand Name: PROPION VAGINAL GEL**
- **Manufacturer:** Wyeth
- **Use:** Vaginal fungal infection
- **Dosage Form:** Gel
- **Administration:** Vaginal
- **Ingredients:** Calcium propionate 10%, sodium propionate 10%, boric acid 3% (antifungals).

PROPION GEL is used to treat fungal infections of the vulvovaginal area. A number of effective preparations exist for treating vaginal infections of fungal origin, such as topically-applied nystatin. Boric acid, one of the active ingredients in Propion Gel, is a weak acid. Even at 3 percent concentration, boric acid inhibits bacterial growth but does not destroy many forms of bacteria. According to *AMA Drug Evaluations* (second edition, pg. 653), "boric acid has no useful place in modern medicine." How much boric acid is absorbed through normal application of Propion Gel is unknown, but it could be significant.

- **Brand Name: PROTERNOL**
- **Manufacturer:** Key
- **Use:** Heartblock and Stokes-Adams Syndrome
- **Dosage Form:** Time-release tablet
- **Administration:** Oral
- **Ingredients:** Isoproterenol hydrochloride 15 or 30 mg (adrenergic/stimulant).

PROTERNOL, an adrenalin-like drug, is used to treat heart block (an abnormality in the conduction of normal electrical impulses through the heart, causing a slow pulse and sometimes episodes of dizziness or fainting).

Isoproterenol has been demonstrated to be effective when used intravenously. It acts to speed the heart rate, increase the force of heart beats, dilate blood vessels and relax the bronchial passages. However, thus far Proternol, marketed in time-release oral form, has been lacking in convincing evidence of efficacy. Studies show that this drug is largely inactivated by the liver when taken in oral form, and thus doesn't become available in sufficient quantities at the desired site of action, the heart. However, this issue is still the subject of ongoing research.

- **Brand Name: QUADRINAL**
- **Manufacturer:** Knoll
- **Use:** Asthma, respiratory disorders
- **Dosage Form:** Tablet
- **Administration:** Oral
- **Ingredients:** Ephedrine hydrochloride 24 mg, theophylline calcium salicylate 130 mg (bronchodilators); phenobarbital 24 mg (sedative); potassium iodide 320 mg (expectorant).

QUADRINAL is a multi-drug combination used to treat chronic respiratory diseases, such as bronchial asthma and chronic bronchitis, in which tenacious mucus and bronchospasm are dominant problems.

Two ingredients included in Quadrinal, ephedrine and theophylline, are effective in relieving asthmatic symptoms when wheezing and constricted ("tight") air passages are significant problems, though theophylline is present in smaller quantities than is needed by many adults. Moreover, there is some evidence that ephedrine loses its effectiveness when used on a chronic basis. It may also cause or aggravate high blood pressure. Sedatives (phenobarbital) and expectorants (potassium iodide) have not been proven effective in treating asthma. When taken regularly, phenobarbital can also cause physical and psychological addiction.

See similar drug ASMINYL, pg. 51

- **Brand Name: QUIBRON PLUS**
- **Manufacturer:** Mead Johnson
- **Use:** Asthma, respiratory disorders
- **Dosage Form:** Capsule / Elixir
- **Administration:** Oral / Oral
- **Ingredients:** Ephedrine hydrochloride, theophylline (bronchodilators); butabarbital (sedative); guaifenesin (expectorant); alcohol 15% (in elixir).

QUIBRON PLUS is used to treat chronic respiratory diseases, such as asthma and chronic bronchitis, in which tenacious mucus and constricted bronchial (breathing) passages are important problems.

Two of the ingredients, ephedrine and theophylline, are useful in relieving asthmatic symptoms of wheezing and constricted ("tight") air passages. However, theophylline must be used in the proper individualized dose and the small dose in Quibron Plus may not be effective for many people. Ephedrine loses its effectiveness when used regularly and can cause or aggravate high blood pressure. The efficacy of sedatives (butabarbital) and expectorants (guaifenesin) in asthma and related disorders is not documented. When taken on a regular basis, butabarbital may also lead to both psychological and physical addiction.

- **Brand Name: RAUTRAX**
- **Manufacturer:** Squibb
- **Use:** High blood pressure
- **Dosage Form:** Tablet
- **Administration:** Oral
- **Ingredients:** Flumethiazide 400 mg (diuretic); rauwolfia (Raudixin) 50 mg (antihypertensive); potassium chloride 400 mg (salt).

RAUTRAX is a combination product used to treat high blood pressure. It contains the effective blood pressure-lowering drug rauwolfia (a form of reserpine) and the useful diuretic (anti-fluid retention drug) flumethiazide. It also includes 400 mg of potassium chloride (KCl), an important mineral. However, the FDA presently considers this product as well as the other two Rautrax products listed in this book (Rautrax-N and Rautrax-N Modified) as failing to meet the standards of effectiveness. These products are examples in which the individual components are effective, but the fixed-combination constitutes an unacceptable medication.

The use of a diuretic drug for high blood pressure is often appropriate. Since most diuretics lower the body's level of potassium, potassium supplementation is often necessary. Squibb, therefore, produces three Rautrax drugs which contain fixed amounts of potassium salt and claims that this alleviates the problem of potassium deficiency. The trouble is that in most cases it is unlikely that Rautrax would supply enough extra potassium to make up for the loss. The combination may create a false sense of security that could allow a potassium deficiency to develop. What is more, some people may not need the potassium or may even be harmed by it. Thus Rautrax suffers from the common problem of fixed-combination products: therapy cannot be tailored to the individual patient's needs. In addition, potassium salts found in tablets or capsules, such as Rautrax, have caused serious intestinal ulcers, so that additional potassium should always be given in dietary supplements and solution form. Finally, it is much cheaper for a patient to buy potassium separately (in liquid form or purchased as a tablet or powder and made into a liquid) than as part of a prescription drug fixed-combination. Potassium supplementation should be carefully monitored by one's physician if it has been determined that such therapy is indeed necessary. For reasons of safety and effectiveness as well as cost, Rautrax should be avoided.

Each of the Rautrax fixed-combination products also contains a second-line antihypertensive agent, rauwolfia (Raudixin) containing reserpine. Until 1974, reserpine was considered fairly safe and effective for treating high blood pressure that was not adequately controlled by weight loss, reducing salt intake, and the use of a diuretic drug (water pill). However, in 1974, three important medical studies were published that linked reserpine to the development of breast cancer in women. The studies had been conducted independently in Boston, England and Finland, and each discovered an increased incidence of cancer in women taking reserpine -containing medications.[1]

Apparently this evidence was not persuasive enough to merit the restriction of this drug, for it is still prescribed in large quantities. However, in 1979, scientists at the National Cancer Institute (NCI) reported that laboratory animals had developed cancer after exposure to reserpine. While reserpine must be regarded as probably carcinogenic for humans, an NCI spokesman said, "the extent of the risk that might be posed by commonly used dosages of the drug cannot be established."[2] "Even if the question of cancer had not arisen, there is still some doubt that reserpine should be considered a primary agent for the treatment of high blood pressure."[3]

Reserpine produces a high incidence of unpleasant side effects. Drowsiness, diarrhea, nausea, sedation, fatigue, stomach ulceration, slow heartbeat, nasal congestion, muscle stiffness, nightmares and psychological depression are only some of the more common adverse reactions associated with reserpine.[4] According to an article in the *New England Journal of Medicine,* "The high frequency of depressive reactions that may be insidious and easily rationalized or passed unnoticed both by the patient and his physician make rauwolfia alkaloids [reserpine] less desirable than oral diuretics for long-term treatment of hypertension."[5]

It has been said that the risk to life posed by untreated high blood pressure "far exceeds" reserpine's potential cancer risk to humans.[6] However, because many other drugs are available that may control high blood pressure, and because reserpine offers few advantages over other second-line drugs, it would appear that its use is not justified except in special situations where all of the safer and more effective alternatives (both non-drug and drug) have been exhausted.

One should remember that most reserpine-containing drug products are considered effective by the FDA. Combination blood-pressure drugs such as Rautrax, however, are considered less than effective because of the questionable efficacy (and safety) of potassium chloride supplements and the questionable effectiveness of mixing rauwolfia and flumethiazide in a rigid formulation. The three Rautrax drugs cited in this text have never been rated higher than ineffective as fixed-combinations by the FDA. They are also the subject of an ongoing safety review. For the treatment of high blood pressure there are effective (and safer) alternatives available.

[1] Boston Collaborative Drug Surveillance Program. *Lancet* 2(7882): 669-671, 1974; Armstrong B, et al. *Lancet* 2(7882): 672-675, 1974; Heinonen O., et al. *Lancet* 2(7882): 675-677, 1974.
[2] *New York Times,* p. A12, May 1, 1979.
[3] Graedon J. *The People's Pharmacy,* 269, 1976.
[4] *Ibid.*
[5] Page LB, et al. *New Eng J Med* 287: 1018-1022, 1972.
[6] *New York Times,* p. A12, May 1, 1979.

- **Brand Name: RAUTRAX-N**
- **Manufacturer:** Squibb
- **Use:** High blood pressure
- **Dosage Form:** Tablet
- **Administration:** Oral
- **Ingredients:** Rauwolfia (Raudixin) 50 mg (antihypertensive); bendroflumethiazide 4 mg (diuretic); potassium chloride 400 mg (salt).

RAUTRAX-N is a fixed-combination product used in the treatment of high blood pressure. Except for the inclusion of a different "thiazide" diuretic (promoting water and salt loss) agent, Rautrax-N is the same as Rautrax, another Squibb product.

Rauwolfia (Raudixin) contains reserpine. Drowsiness, diarrhea, nausea, sedation, fatigue, stomach ulceration, slow heartbeat, nasal congestion, muscle stiffness, nightmares and psychological depression are some of the more common adverse reactions associated with reserpine. In addition, medical studies have linked reserpine to the development of breast cancer in women.

See similar drug RAUTRAX, pg. 165

- **Brand Name: RAUTRAX-N MODIFIED**
- **Manufacturer:** Squibb
- **Use:** High blood pressure
- **Dosage Form:** Tablet
- **Administration:** Oral
- **Ingredients:** Bendroflumethiazide 2 mg (diuretic); rauwolfia (Raudixin) 50 mg (antihypertensive); potassium chloride 400 mg (salt).

RAUTRAX-N MODIFIED is the same as Rautrax-N except this version has 2 mg of the bendroflumethiazide instead of 4 mg.

Rauwolfia (Raudixin) contains reserpine. Drowsiness, diarrhea, nausea, sedation, fatigue, stomach ulceration, slow heartbeat, nasal congestion, muscle stiffness, nightmares and psychological depression are some of the more common adverse reactions associated with reserpine. In addition, medical studies have linked reserpine to the development of breast cancer in women.

See similar drug RAUTRAX-N, pg. 167

- **Brand Name: REPAN**
- **Manufacturer:** Everett
- **Use:** Pain relief
- **Dosage Form:** Tablet
- **Administration:** Oral
- **Ingredients:** Butalbital 50 mg (sedative); caffeine 40 mg (stimulant); phenacetin 130 mg, acetaminophen 300 mg (analgesics).

REPAN is a multi-drug combination prescribed for the relief of pain associated with a variety of conditions. The sedative, butalbital (a barbiturate with addiction potential), allegedly enhances the analgesic effectiveness of this product, providing relief of muscle spasm or relief from anxiety accompanying pain. However, very few properly controlled studies have been designed to find patients who may benefit from mixtures of this sort or to prove that such formulations do, in fact, provide greater symptomatic benefit than acetaminophen alone. If a sedative is needed, it should be administered separately rather than in a fixed-ratio combination. Moreover, there is no convincing evidence that the combination of phenacetin, caffeine and acetaminophen is more effective than acetaminophen alone. Phenacetin causes kidney damage, and reports now suggest that prolonged use of this drug may result in renal cancer and tumors of the nose and urinary tract *(Science,* 204: 4389, 129-130, 1979).

Repan has never been rated higher than "possibly effective" as a fixed-combination by the FDA, and is currently considered lacking in substantial evidence of efficacy.

For the relief of mild to moderate pain, one would do best with simple aspirin or acetaminophen.

- **Brand Name: ROBINUL-PH**
- **Manufacturer:** Robins
- **Use:** Digestive disorders
- **Dosage Form:** Tablet
- **Administration:** Oral
- **Ingredients:** Glycopyrrolate 1 mg (antispasmodic/antisecretory); phenobarbital 16.2 mg (sedative).

ROBINUL-PH is a combination of an antispasmodic/antisecretory agent and a sedative. It is used as back-up therapy in the treatment of stomach ulcer, irritable bowel syndrome and other gastrointestinal disorders.

There is no clinical proof that such mixtures hasten healing of ulcers or prevent their recurrence. Nor is there satisfactory evidence that this combination has any beneficial effect in ulcer patients beyond that afforded by an antacid or antispasmodic/antisecretory agent alone in proper dosage.

The FDA considers plain glycopyrrolate (Robinul) as effective, but only as back-up therapy for ulcer patients and not for those with irritable bowel syndrome. What is at issue here is whether there is satisfactory evidence that the addition of fixed amounts of sedatives to antispasmodic/antisecretory components confers significant therapeutic value to the patient. When taken regularly, phenobarbital can lead to psychological and physical addiction. Glycopyrrolate often causes blurring of vision, dryness of the mouth and throat, constipation and hesitancy of urination.

Also see Part II: Drugs for Digestive Disorders

- **Brand Name: ROBINUL-PH FORTE**
- **Manufacturer:** Robins
- **Use:** Digestive disorders
- **Dosage Form:** Tablet
- **Administration:** Oral
- **Ingredients:** Glycopyrrolate 2 mg (antispasmodic/antisecretory); phenobarbital 16.2 mg (sedative).

ROBINUL-PH FORTE differs from Robinul-PH only in that it includes twice the amount of the antispasmodic/antisecretory agent glycopyrrolate. When taken regularly, phenobarbital can lead to psychological and physical addiction. Glycopyrrolate often causes blurring of vision, dryness of the mouth and throat, constipation and hesitancy of urination.

See similar drug ROBINUL-PH, pg. 169

Also see Part II: Drugs for Digestive Disorders

- **Brand Name: RONIACOL**
- **Manufacturer:** Roche
- **Use:** Blood vessel disease (head and limbs)
- **Dosage Form:** Tablet / Elixir
- **Administration:** Oral / Oral
- **Ingredients:** Nicotinyl alcohol (vasodilator).

RONIACOL is a vasodilator used to treat a variety of conditions associated with deficient blood circulation, such as peripheral vascular disease, varicose ulcers, vascular spasms, a disease of the inner ear (Meniere's Syndrome), and vertigo. Roniacol lacks adequate evidence of clinical efficacy for its labeled indications. Studies using Roniacol have not shown a consistent increase in skin or muscle blood flow in patients with obstructive arterial disease. In fact, a decrease in skin and muscle blood flow during exercise,[1] after exercise and during reactive hyperemia[2] (increased blood flow in a particular part of the body) may occur with the use of this drug product. Thus, Roniacol may even aggravate a case of peripheral artery disease.

In a recent article the author states that "there is no basis for the use of these drugs [nicotinyl alcohol, nicotinic acid] in peripheral vascular diseases."[3] Roniacol has been designated by the FDA as lacking substantial evidence of efficacy. Identical drugs include: Speniacol

[1] Zetterquist S. *Acta Med Scand* 183: 487-496, 1968.
[2] Hansteen V. *Acta Med Scand* [Suppl.] 556: 1-62, 1974.
[3] Coffman JD. *New Eng J Med* 300(13): 713-717, 1979.

Also see Part II: Drugs for Circulatory Disorders of Head and Limbs

- Brand Name: **RONIACOL TIMESPAN TABS**
- **Manufacturer:** Roche
- **Use:** Blood vessel disease (head and limbs)
- **Dosage Form:** Time-release tablet
- **Administration:** Oral
- **Ingredients:** Nicotinyl tartrate 150 mg (vasodilator).

RONIACOL TIMESPAN TABS are comprised of a tartrate salt of nicotinyl alcohol in a time-release form and have the same labeled indications as Roniacol. There is no evidence that this is a useful therapeutic agent for peripheral vascular disorders, and it is presently considered lacking in substantial evidence of efficacy.

See similar drug RONIACOL, pg. 170

Also see Part II: Drugs for Circulatory Disorders of Head and Limbs

- **Brand Name: RU-VERT**
- **Manufacturer:** Boots
- **Use:** Central nervous system stimulation
- **Dosage Form:** Tablet
- **Administration:** Oral
- **Ingredients:** Pentylenetetrazol 25 mg (stimulant/analgesic); niacin (vitamin/vasodilator); pheniramine maleate (antihistamine).

RU-VERT is the most widely prescribed pentylenetetrazol-containing combination drug. Its manufacturer promotes Ru-Vert for vertigo, but this drug and others like it are commonly used as central nervous system stimulants to treat the elderly for a wide variety of symptoms including senile confusion and depression. However, all these drugs are ineffective, irrational and potentially dangerous. Pheniramine can cause drowsiness, loss of coordination, mental inattention and dizziness. Pentylenetetrazol was once the mainstay for treating the cessation of breathing (apnea) and drug-induced coma. However, according to *AMA Drug Evaluations* (second edition, pg. 279) this drug "should no longer be used." These ineffective drugs may be likened to the old-time tonics and panaceas; they provide no benefit to the patient and should be pulled from the market.

- **Brand Name: SIDONNA**
- **Manufacturer:** Reed and Carnick
- **Use:** Digestive disorders
- **Dosage Form:** Tablet
- **Administration:** Oral
- **Ingredients:** Hyoscyamine sulfate .1037 mg, atropine sulfate .0194 mg, hyoscine hydrobromide .0065 mg, (antispasmodic/antisecretories); sodium butabarbital 16 mg (sedative); simethicone 25 mg (gas dispenser).

SIDONNA is promoted as back-up therapy in the treatment of irritable bowel syndrome and acute inflammation of the intestines and colon. This drug suffers from all the disadvantages commonly associated with fixed-combination drugs. The antispasmodic/antisecretory drugs in Sidonna are all present in amounts that are too small to provide any real therapeutic benefit. In addition the fact that five separate drugs are in this product almost assures that the relative amounts of each drug will not be optimum for any given situation. When taken regularly, butabarbital can lead to psychological and physical addiction. Hyoscyamine, atropine and hyoscine often cause blurring of vision, dryness of the mouth and throat, constipation and hesitancy of urination.

See similar drug DONNATAL, pg. 93

Also see Part II: Drugs for Digestive Disorders

- Brand Name: **SPECTROCIN**
- **Manufacturer:** Squibb
- **Use:** Skin disorders
- **Dosage Form:** Ointment
- **Administration:** Topical
- **Ingredients:** Neomycin sulfate 3.6 mg, gramicidin 0.25 mg (antibacterials) per gram.

SPECTROCIN, a fixed-combination topical ointment, is prescribed for a wide variety of skin disorders involving infection or the threat of infection. It is also available without a prescription. Its uses include treatment of biopsy sites, skin ulcers and boils, minor burns, abrasions, cuts, infected eczema and related skin problems, such as impetigo. Spectrocin is also administered as a preventive measure when the skin has been broken due to a cut or burn.

The use of topical antibiotics like those contained in Spectrocin is, at best, debatable. In addition to their lack of efficacy these drugs may cause skin rashes, allergic reactions and sensitivity to other more important antibiotics.

Also see Part II: Drugs Applied Directly to Skin, Eye or Ear

- Brand Name: **SPENTANE T.D.**
- **Manufacturer:** Spencer-Mead
- **Use:** Cold and allergy
- **Dosage Form:** Time-release tablet
- **Administration:** Oral
- **Ingredients:** Brompheniramine maleate 8 or 12 mg (antihistamine).

SPENTANE T.D. is promoted for seasonal hay fever and nasal congestion, as well as other allergic conditions. This product is both chemically and pharmacologically very similar to chlorpheniramine.

If one needs an antihistamine, one should use generic chlorpheniramine maleate (2 or 4 mg). For this product, it is the "long-lasting" dosage form that is of questionable value, not the drug ingredient itself. Its use is generally not recommended because of uneven action. Brompheniramine can cause drowsiness, loss of coordination, mental inattention and dizziness. Identical drugs include: Bromatane, Brompheniramine Maleate, Puretane.

Also see Part II: Drugs for Cough, Cold and Allergy.

- **Brand Name: SULFATHALIDINE**
- **Manufacturer:** Merck, Sharpe and Dohme
- **Use:** Inflammatory bowel disease
- **Dosage Form:** Tablet
- **Administration:** Oral
- **Ingredients:** Phthalylsulfathiazole 500 mg (anti-infective).

SULFATHALIDINE is an anti-infective drug used as an adjunct in the long-term management of bowel disease and in the pre-operative preparation of patients undergoing bowel surgery. This drug is not considered effective for these disorders. Sulfa drugs such as phthalylsulfathiazole can cause allergic reactions, headache, dizziness, nausea, vomiting and, rarely, serious blood disorders. Inflammatory bowel disease is a severe, usually chronic condition, which may require surgery and may progress despite all therapy.

- **Brand Name: SYNALGOS**
- **Manufacturer:** Ives
- **Use:** Pain relief
- **Dosage Form:** Capsule
- **Administration:** Oral
- **Ingredients:** Promethazine hydrochloride 6.25 mg (antihistamine/sedative); phenacetin 162 mg (analgesic); aspirin 194 mg (analgesic/antipyretic); caffeine 30 mg (stimulant).

SYNALGOS is a multi-drug combination prescribed for the relief of mild to moderate pain and related nervousness associated with a variety of conditions. There is no convincing evidence that promethazine, an antihistamine-like drug belonging to the phenothiazine (as in Thorazine) class, with sedative and anti-nausea properties, contributes to the effectiveness of Synalgos as a pain-relief product.

The possible toxicity of promethazine (jaundice, decreased production of white blood cells, Parkinsonian symptoms and rashes) argues against its use in minor illnesses even if it were effective in conjunction with APC. (See below)

As the *AMA Drug Evaluations* (third edition, pg. 1104) states, promethazine "can produce any of the adverse reactions observed with other phenothiazines." Although none of the phenothiazine drugs (most are sold as tranquilizers) appear to be completely free of the risk of complications affecting the nervous system (extrapyramidal stimulation), which is being recognized more frequently, especially in older patients, "promethazine is relatively free of . . . extrapyramidal stimulation" (Ibid).

While adverse reactions are less likely to happen with only occasional use of promethazine-containing drugs like Synalgos, doctors should realize that the promethazine in these products confers no counterbalancing medical benefit to the patient. Promethazine can also cause drowsiness, loss of coordination, mental inattention and dizziness.

Aspirin, Phenacetin and Caffeine (APC)

This triple combination is one of the most frequently used mixtures of analgesic drugs, and forms the "core" of the Synalgos products. However, as is stated in the *AMA Drug Evaluations* (second edition, pg. 269), "there is no convincing evidence that the rationale for this combination is sound." Since both aspirin and phenacetin have pain relieving and anti-fever properties, "there is no advantage in combining them. Furthermore, since phenacetin has little anti-inflammatory action, the combination would be less effective than an equivalent amount of aspirin alone in treating inflammatory conditions. Although the vascular effect of caffeine [vasoconstriction] may be useful in the treatment of migraine headache, there is no evidence that the small amount contained in the usual APC formulation [40 mg, or less than ½ the amount in a cup of coffee] has an analgesic [pain relieving] effect or that it affects the activity of the analgesic components." Even though APC has been approved for safety and efficacy by the FDA, "there have been no well-controlled studies showing that either phenacetin or APC is more effective than aspirin alone as an analgesic."[1] Additionally, phenacetin is known to cause kidney damage and is thought to be a carcinogen.[2]

[1] *The Medical Letter* 8: 2, Jan. 28, 1966.
[2] Tomatis, L. *Science* 204: 4389, 129-130, 1979.

- **Brand Name: SYNALGOS-DC**
- **Manufacturer:** Ives
- **Use:** Pain relief
- **Dosage Form:** Capsule
- **Administration:** Oral
- **Ingredients:** Promethazine hydrochloride 6.25 mg (antihistamine/sedative); phenacetin 162 mg (analgesic); dihydrocodeine bitartrate 16 mg (analgesic/narcotic); aspirin 194 mg (analgesic/antipyretic); caffeine 30 mg (stimulant).

SYNALGOS-DC is a fixed-combination product prescribed for the relief of moderate to moderately severe pain and related anxiety associated with a variety of conditions.

Dihydrocodeine bitartrate is a drug with proven pain relieving properties and, when used correctly, can play a useful medical role. However, the other components of this mixture have little or no value in the relief of moderate to severe pain.* There is no evidence that promethazine contributes to dihydrocodeine in relieving pain. The FDA has classified this product as lacking substantial evidence of effectiveness. Promethazine can cause drowsiness, loss of coordination, mental inattention and dizziness. Phenacetin can cause kidney damage, kidney cancer and tumors of the nose and urinary tract.

See SYNALGOS, pg. 174, identical to SYNALGOS-DC but without the DC (dihydrocodeine bitartrate)

*Aspirin alone is effective for minor to moderate pain.

- **Brand Name: TARCORTIN**
- **Manufacturer:** Reed and Carnrick
- **Use:** Skin disorders
- **Dosage Form:** Cream
- **Administration:** Topical
- **Ingredients:** Hydrocortisone .5% (corticosteroid); crude coal tar 5% (antieczematic).

TARCORTIN is a combination corticosteroid-tar product prescribed for the treatment of a variety of acute and chronic skin conditions, such as allergic eczema, psoriasis and seborrhea. According to *AMA Drug Evaluations* (second edition, pg. 908), coal tar has a tendency to produce skin irritation, although this appears to be negligible in patients with psoriasis. Coal tar has been known to precipitate severe skin reactions and occasionally is photosensiti-

zing. For safety as well as economy, it is sensible to use a simple generic hydrocortisone cream if a steroid is indicated.

Also see Part II: Drugs Applied Directly to Skin, Eye or Ear

- Brand Name: **TELDRIN**
- **Manufacturer:** Smith Kline & French
- **Use:** Cold and allergy
- **Dosage Form:** Time-release capsule
- **Administration:** Oral
- **Ingredients:** Chlorpheniramine maleate 8 or 12 mg (antihistamine).

TELDRIN is used for the treatment of hay fever and other allergic conditions. The time-release capsule dosage forms (8 or 12 mg) are not recommended because their longer action is uneven and their additional cost is unnecessary.

In this case, the time-release formulation, rather than the drug itself, is of unproven efficacy. Chlorpheniramine, when given in its usual 4 mg dosage, is an effective, relatively inexpensive medicine for treating allergic conditions, such as hay fever and hives. There is no convincing evidence, however, that it provides any benefit in treating colds. Teldrin is now available without a prescription. Chlorpheniramine can cause drowsiness, loss of coordination, mental inattention and dizziness. Identical drugs include: Allerid-O.D.-8, Allerid-O.D.-12, Chloramate Unicelles, Chlorophen, Chlorpheniramine Maleate(8 or 12 mg), Chlorspan 12, Histaspan, Histex, Histrey, Phenetron Lanacaps, T.D. Alermine, Trymegen Time-sules.

Also see Part II: Drugs for Cough, Cold and Allergy

- **Brand Name: TERRA-CORTRIL OPHTHALMIC**
- **Manufacturer:** Pfizer
- **Use:** Eye infection, inflammation
- **Dosage Form:** Suspension
- **Administration:** Eye
- **Ingredients:** Oxytetracycline hydrochloride 0.5% (antibacterial); hydrocortisone acetate 1.5% (corticosteroid).

TERRA-CORTRIL OPHTHALMIC is prescribed for various eye and eyelid infections of bacterial and allergic origin, as well as a number of non-specific inflammatory conditions. The use of topical antibiotics is at best debatable. The use of corticosteroids for the treatment of eye infections may be dangerous because they can either mask the evidence of infection or cause the spreading of infections.

Also see Part II: Drugs Applied Directly to Skin, Eye or Ear

- **Brand Name: TERRA-CORTRIL TOPICAL**
- **Manufacturer:** Pfizer
- **Use:** Skin infection
- **Dosage Form:** Ointment
- **Administration:** Topical
- **Ingredients:** Oxytetracycline hydrochloride 3% (antibacterial); hydrocortisone 1% (corticosteroid).

TERRA-CORTRIL TOPICAL is prescribed for skin infections, including those due to wounds and minor burns, various skin diseases (allergic eczema, contact dermatitis), and non-specific itching (pruritus) of the anus, vulva and scrotum.

The use of corticosteroids for the treatment of skin infections may be dangerous because they can either mask the evidence of infection or cause the spreading of infections. Antibacterial agents should not be used in the treatment of non-infectious skin disorders, and their use for skin infections is also highly questionable.

If infections are present in wounds and antibiotics are needed, they should probably be given orally or by injection. Wounds, if properly cleaned with soap and water, usually do well by themselves. Antibiotic-corticosteroid mixtures should be avoided.

Also see Part II: Drugs Applied Directly to Skin, Eye or Ear

- Brand Name: **TERRASTATIN**
- **Manufacturer:** Pfizer
- **Use:** Bacterial and fungal infection
- **Dosage Form:** Capsule
- **Administration:** Oral
- **Ingredients:** Oxytetracycline 250 mg (antibacterial); nystatin 250,000 u (antifungal); glucosamine hydrochloride 250 mg (sugar).

TERRASTATIN is a fixed-combination drug product prescribed to eliminate a wide variety of infections of bacterial and fungal origin, e.g., pneumonia, other respiratory tract infections, genitourinary infections, eye infections, surgical infections and gastrointestinal infections. The antifungal agent, nystatin, is added to prevent fungal overgrowth, certainly a rare clinical entity during drug therapy with tetracyclines and other antibiotics.

According to the *AMA Drug Evaluations* (third edition, p. 752), it is preferable to administer nystatin on an individual basis when dual therapy with a broad spectrum antibiotic is considered desirable. Nystatin may cause transient nausea and vomiting after oral administration. Also, the addition of glucosamine, a type of sugar, confers no therapeutic benefit to the patient.

See similar drug MYSTECLIN F, pg. 122

- **Brand Name: THERAPAV**
- **Manufacturer:** Cooper
- **Use:** Blood vessel disease (head and limbs)
- **Dosage Form:** Liquid filled capsule
- **Administration:** Oral
- **Ingredients:** Papaverine hydrochloride 75 or 150 mg (vasodilator).

THERAPAV is a papaverine-based drug product usually

prescribed for disorders due to insufficient blood flow to the head and limbs. Less frequently, it is used for pain due to insufficient blood flow to the heart. Papaverine products are used primarily with elderly patients.

There is currently no evidence that any papaverine product is effective for its recommended uses, and there is strong evidence that these products can cause liver damage in many people. *(New Eng J Med* 281: 1333-35 and 1364-65, 1969)

See similar drug PAPAVERINE, pg. 143

Also see Part II: Drugs for Circulatory Disorders of Head and Limbs

- **Brand Name: TIGAN RECTAL SUPPOSITORIES**
- **Manufacturer:** Beecham
- **Use:** Nausea and vomiting
- **Dosage Form:** Suppository
- **Administration:** Rectal
- **Ingredients:** Trimethobenzamide hydrochloride 100 or 200 mg (antiemetic).

TIGAN SUPPOSITORIES are promoted for

the control of nausea and vomiting. The mechanism of action of this drug as determined in animals is obscure, but the drug is claimed to inhibit the vomiting center of the brain. The FDA has recently reclassified this drug product as lacking substantial evidence of effectiveness for its labeled indications and has initiated the procedure required to remove the drug from the market. However, Tigan Suppositories are still readily available.

In 1977, Beecham Laboratories submitted results of studies to the

FDA which verified that the suppository form of Tigan is not "bio-equivalent" to the injectable dosage form. This means the drug is not adequately released and absorbed by the body in this rectal suppository form, and sufficient blood levels are not obtained.

Furthermore, the FDA stated that adequate clinical studies of this product's efficacy have not been conducted.

- **Brand Name: TROCINATE**
- **Manufacturer:** Poythress
- **Use:** Digestive disorders
- **Dosage Form:** Tablet
- **Administration:** Oral
- **Ingredients:** Thiphenamil hydrochloride 100 or 400 mg (antispasmodic).

TROCINATE is a single-entity drug prescribed for relief of the pain and discomfort due to smooth muscle spasm associated with irritable bowel syndrome and a variety of functional gastrointestinal disorders. The active ingredient of Trocinate, thiphenamil, lacks evidence of effectiveness for the treatment of these symptoms. Belladonna or atropine, available generically, are effective. Thiphenamil often causes blurring of vision, dryness of the mouth and throat, constipation and hesitancy of urination.

Also see Part II: Drugs for Digestive Disorders

- **Brand Name: TUSSIONEX**
- **Manufacturer:** Pennwalt
- **Use:** Cough and cold
- **Dosage form:** Tablet /Syrup/ Capsule
- **Administration:** Oral/ Oral/ Oral
- **Ingredients:** Hydrocodone (antitussive/narcotic); phenyltoloxamine (antihistamine).

TUSSIONEX is a fixed-combination drug product promoted for the suppression of cough. An antihistamine, phenyltoloxamine, is blended with hydrocodone. However, there is no convincing evidence that it augments the cough-suppressing action of hydrocodone in any way. In fact, antihistamines have the effect of thickening bronchial secretions and may actually create problems for patients who produce mucus with their coughs or who have difficulty breathing. Although there is ample evidence that hydrocodone is an effective cough suppressant, it also has a great dependence liability. The National Academy of Sciences-National Research Council rated this drug ineffective as a fixed-combination. If a drug remedy is considered necessary for a cough, plain generic dextromethorphan (non-narcotic) is the best therapy. Phenyltoloxamine can cause drowsiness, loss of coordination, mental inattention and dizziness.

Also see Part II: Drugs for Cough, Cold and Allergy

- **Brand Name: TUSS-ORNADE**
- **Manufacturer:** Smith Kline & French
- **Use:** Cough, cold, allergy
- **Dosage Form:** Time-release capsule / Liquid
- **Administration:** Oral   / Oral
- **Ingredients:** Caramiphen edisylate (antitussive); isopropamide iodide (anticholinergic); chlorpheniramine maleate (antihistamine); phenylpropanolamine hydrochloride (sympathomimetic).

TUSS-ORNADE is a pharmaceutical potpourri used for relief from coughing, upper respiratory congestion and the symptoms associated with the common cold and allergic nasal conditions. This product is one of a number of ineffective "shotgun" approaches to treating cough and cold symptoms. There is a lack of substantial clinical evidence of efficacy for this mixture. It is composed of an antitussive agent, an anticholinergic, an antihistamine and a sympathomimetic. However, none of the four ingredients has proven cough-suppressing properties, and antihistamines are of no value in treating the common cold. Because of its variable absorption and uneven course of action, the time-release capsule form would be unacceptable even if all four ingredients made effective contributions. For congestion due to allergy, a single antihistamine such as chlorpheniramine maleate is recommended. If a cough needs to be treated with drug therapy, then dextromethorphan should be used. (Productive cough with phlegm should not be treated, as it is the body's way of ridding itself of secretions and guarding against infection.) Tuss-Ornade has been rated ineffective by the FDA as a fixed-combination for all of its labeled indications. Isopropamide often causes blurring of vision, dryness of the mouth and throat, constipation and hesitancy of urination. Phenylpropanolamine can cause or aggravate high blood pressure and commonly loses its effectiveness when used regularly. Chlorpheniramine can cause drowsiness, loss of coordination, mental inattention and dizziness. Identical drugs include: Tuss-Ade Liquid, Tusscaps, Tuss-Liquid.

Also see Part II: Drugs for Cough, Cold and Allergy.

- **Brand Name: UROBIOTIC-250**
- **Manufacturer:** Roerig
- **Use:** Genitourinary tract infection
- **Dosage Form:** Capsule
- **Administration:** Oral
- **Ingredients:** Oxytetracycline hydrochloride 250 mg, sulfamethizole 250 mg (antibacterials); phenazopyridine hydrochloride 50 mg (urinary tract analgesic).

UROBIOTIC-250 is prescribed for the treatment of a number of genitourinary tract (G.U.) infections caused by organisms susceptible to the antibacterials included in this drug mixture. This drug product combines two antibacterial agents with phenazopyridine, a drug which produces local pain relief in the G.U. tract.

Since no additive action has been demonstrated between the two components (oxytetracycline and sulfamethizole), the use of either agent alone is preferred, although sulfamethizole is usually the more appropriate drug. Moreover, there is no persuasive evidence that the addition of phenazopyridine confers any significant therapeutic benefit to the patient.

Urinary tract infections can usually be treated with single-entity drugs. Although there are other equally effective antibiotics available for treating these infections, the so-called short-acting sulfonamide drug family is often prescribed. The specific agents in this group are excreted into the urinary tract in high antibacterial concentration (largely in the active form) and maintain adequate drug levels in the blood and tissues during the period of urinary excretion. Since the infection is localized in the bladder and urinary tract, this action is quite desirable. Sulfamethizole (Thiosulfil) and sulfisoxazole (Gantrisin) are two of the most useful drugs in this class.

Sulfamethizole (and other sulfonamide drugs) can often produce hypersensitivity reactions affecting the skin and mucous membranes. These reactions are of the allergic type and include itching and rash. Nausea and vomiting have been frequently reported with the use of these drugs. More rarely, sulfamethizole may also cause blood disorders. Nystatin can cause nausea and vomiting.

- Brand Name: **VALPIN 50-PB**
- **Manufacturer:** Endo
- **Use:** Digestive disorders
- **Dosage Form:** Tablet
- **Administration:** Oral
- **Ingredients:** Anisotropine methylbromide 50 mg (antispasmodic/antisecretory); phenobarbital 15 mg (sedative).

VALPIN is prescribed to treat peptic ulcer, irritable bowel syndrome and other gastrointestinal conditions. Valpin 50-PB is one of many drugs cited in this book that contain an antispasmodic/ antisecretory agent in combination with a fixed amount of a sedative. There is still a lack of adequate clinical evidence to support the claim that adding a sedative to an antispasmodic/antisecretory drug in a rigid fixed-ratio confers significant therapeutic benefit to the patient. When taken regularly phenobarbital can lead to psychological and physical addiction. Anisotropine methylbromide often causes blurring of vision, dryness of the mouth and throat, constipation and hesitancy of urination.

Also see Part II: Drugs for Digestive Disorders

- **Brand Name: VASOCON-A**
- **Manufacturer:** Smith, Miller & Patch
- **Use:** Allergic eye disorders
- **Dosage Form:** Solution
- **Administration:** Eye
- **Ingredients:** Naphazoline hydrochloride 0.05% (decongestant); antazoline phosphate 0.5% (antihistamine); boric acid 1.2% (antiseptic); phenylmercuric acetate 0.002% (preservative).

VASOCON-A is a fixed-combination product containing the decongestant naphazoline and the antihistamine antazoline. It is advocated for the treatment of allergic eye disorders. Topically applied antihistamines, however, are quite ineffective in combating allergic reactions. Any symptomatic relief obtained from Vasocon-A is probably due to the local anesthetic properties of the antazoline phosphate and possibly to the vasoconstrictor action of the naphazoline decongestant. For patients who have become sensitized to the antihistamine in Vasocon-A, the subsequent oral administration of an antihistamine or a chemically related drug for a general allergic condition may cause an eczematous type of allergic reaction. Identical drugs include: Albalon-A Liquifilm.

Also see Part II: Drugs Applied Directly to Skin, Eye or Ear

- **Brand Name: VASODILAN**
- **Manufacturer:** Mead Johnson
- **Use:** Blood vessel disease (head and limbs)
- **Dosage Form:** Tablet /Solution
- **Administration:** Oral/ Injection
- **Ingredients:** Isoxsuprine hydrochloride (vasodilator).

VASODILAN, a direct-acting blood vessel dilator, is sold and prescribed for the relief of symptoms associated with insufficient blood flow to the brain tissue and a variety of obstructive peripheral blood vessel disorders. Since it is not a dilator of skin blood vessels, it is not indicated in disorders characterized by vasospasm (spastic vessel constriction) such as Raynaud's disease. As with most of the peripheral and cerebro-vasodilators used today, there is a lack of substantial clinical evidence of efficacy for Vasodilan. In a recent article, the author states that "studies do not support the use of this drug in obstructive arterial disease," its principal usage (*New Eng. J. Med.* 300: 713-717, 1979). Identical drugs include: Isoxsuprine HCl, Vasoprine.

Also see Part II: Drugs for Circulatory Disorders of Head and Limbs

- Brand Name: **VIOFORM-HYDROCORTISONE**
- **Manufacturer:** Ciba
- **Use:** Skin disorders
- **Dosage Form:** Ointment /Cream /Lotion
- **Administration:** Topical / Topical/ Topical
- **Ingredients:** Iodochlorhydroxyquin 3% (anti-infective); hydrocortisone 1% (corticosteroid).

VIOFORM-HYDROCORTISONE is
promoted and prescribed for the treatment of a wide variety of skin conditions involving fungal (yeast) infection, bacterial infection, and/or inflammatory manifestations. If fungal infection is present, one should use an effective antifungal agent, such as nystatin or amphotericin B. The use of corticosteroids for the treatment of skin infections may be dangerous because they can either mask the evidence of infection or cause the spreading of infections. If hydrocortisone is needed for skin conditions not of fungal/bacterial origin, it should nearly always be administered by itself under close medical supervision.

Identical drugs include: Caquin, Cortin, Durel-Cort V, Epiform-HC, Hydrocortisone w/Iodochlorhydroxyquin, Hysone, Iodocort, Lanvisone, Oxyquin, Pedi-Cort-V, Vio-Hydrocort, Vioquin HC, Viotag.

Also see Part II: Drugs Applied Directly to Skin, Eye or Ear

- **Brand Name:** VIOFORM-HYDROCORTISONE MILD
- **Manufacturer:** Ciba
- **Use:** Skin disorders
- **Dosage Form:** Ointment /Cream
- **Administration:** Topical / Topical
- **Ingredients:** Iodochlorhydroxyquin 3% (anti-infective); hydrocortisone 0.5% (corticosteroid).

VIOFORM-HYDROCORTISONE

MILD is identical to the plain form except that its concentration of hydrocortisone, the anti-inflammatory agent, is one-half. The use of corticosteroids for the treatment of skin infections may be dangerous because they can either mask the evidence of infection or cause the spreading of infections. Identical drugs include: Bafil, Cortin, Domeform-HC, Durel-Cort V, Hexaderm I.Q., Hydrocortisone w/Iodochlorhydroxyquin, Mity-Quin, Racet.

See similar drug VIOFORM-HYDROCORTISONE, pg. 186

Also see Part II: Drugs Applied Directly to Skin, Eye or Ear

- **Brand Name:** VITA-METRAZOL
- **Manufacturer:** Knoll
- **Use:** Central nervous system stimulation
- **Dosage Form:** Elixir /Tablet
- **Administration:** Oral/ Oral
- **Ingredients:** Pentylenetetrazol (stimulant/analeptic); vitamins B-1, B-2, niacinamide, B-6, C, (vitamins).

VITA-METRAZOL is a combination of a central nervous system (CNS) stimulant and a collection of vitamins (one with blood vessel dilating properties) administered to enhance the mental and physical activity of elderly patients.

See similar drug RU-VERT, pg. 172

- **Brand Name: VYTONE**
- **Manufacturer:** Dermik
- **Use:** Skin disorders
- **Dosage Form:** Cream
- **Administration:** Topical
- **Ingredients:** Diiodohydroxyquin 1% (anti-infective); hydrocortisone 1% (corticosteroid).

VYTONE is virtually the same as Vioform-Hydrocortisone and is prescribed for the same types of skin disorders, such as bacterial or fungal infections. The use of corticosteroids for the treatment of skin infections may be dangerous because they can either mask the evidence of infection or cause the spreading of infections. Identical drugs include: Cort-Quin.

See similar drug VIOFORM-HYDROCORTISONE, pg. 186

Also see Part II: Drugs Applied Directly to Skin, Eye or Ear

- **Brand Name: WINSTROL**
- **Manufacturer:** Winthrop
- **Use:** Bone, growth disorders
- **Dosage Form:** Tablet
- **Administration:** Oral
- **Ingredients:** Stanozolol 2 mg (androgenic steroid).

WINSTROL, like other weak androgen (male hormone) steroids in its class, is used as adjunctive therapy in the treatment of senile and postmenopausal bone disorders (progressive decrease in total bone mass). It has also been used in children for the management of certain growth disorders but this can result in irreversible adverse effects, such as masculinization of girls. The National Academy of Sciences-National Research Council cautions that these drugs are without value as primary therapy in the treatment of progressive bone disorder (osteoporosis).

Unfortunately, at the present time there are no available prescription drugs considered truly effective in the treatment of osteoporosis. Primary therapy for this bone disease is said to be diet, calcium balance, physiotherapy and general attention to health. (The usual alternative to these weak androgens is conjugated estrogen such as Premarin, which lacks evidence of effectiveness for this indication. Estrogens also carry appreciable risk of developing cancer for postmenopausal women.)

According to the *AMA Drug Evaluations* (second edition, pg. 407), these drugs such as Winstrol have been used in patients recovering from surgery, infections, burns, and fractures, but there is no adequate evidence that their use shortens the period of recovery. It goes on to say that "objective evidence of improvement in patients with senile or corticosteroid-induced osteoporosis has not been demonstrated." Winstrol's side effects also include masculinization of women.

The FDA claims that Winstrol and other androgenic steroids may be used with extreme caution, in selective cases of growth failure, and in patients with pituitary dwarfism (a condition resulting from inadequate bodily production of growth hormone) until growth hormone is commercially available. However, there is a possibility of causing serious disturbances of growth and sexual development if given to young children.

- Brand Name: **WYANOIDS HC RECTAL SUPPOSITORIES**
- **Manufacturer:** Wyeth
- **Use:** Anorectal disorders
- **Dosage Form:** Suppository
- **Administration:** Rectal
- **Ingredients:** Hydrocortisone acetate 10 mg (corticosteroid); belladonna extract 15 mg (anticholinergic); ephedrine sulfate 3 mg (sympathomimetic); zinc oxide, boric acid, bismuth oxyiodide (antiseptics); balsam peru (protectant).

WYANOIDS HC is a combination product used for the symptomatic treatment of a number of anorectal inflammatory conditions, such as hemorrhoids, which are often associated with itching, bleeding and pain. This mixture contains a number of ingredients of highly questionable value. According to the *AMA Drug Evaluations* (third edition, pg. 1087), untoward systemic ("whole body") effects may result from the absorption of hydrocortisone through the anorectal mucous membrane and hypersensitivity reactions with severe skin disorders may occur after the topical application of the several antiseptic ingredients in this preparation. In 1974, the FDA downgraded Wyanoids HC to lacking substantial evidence of effectiveness and offered Wyeth Laboratories, its manufacturer, an opportunity to respond to the FDA proposal to withdraw marketing approval for this product. Identical drugs include: Rectacort Suppositories.

- **Brand Name: ZACTANE**
- **Manufacturer:** Wyeth
- **Use:** Pain relief
- **Dosage Form:** Tablet
- **Administration:** Oral
- **Ingredients:** Ethoheptazine citrate 75 mg (analgesic).

ZACTANE is a drug prescribed and promoted for the relief of mild to moderate pain associated with a number of conditions. It has none of the anti-inflammatory or anti-fever action found in aspirin. Well-controlled clinical studies do not confirm its effectiveness as a pain reliever. The FDA has classified this drug as lacking substantial evidence of effectiveness.

- **Brand Name: ZACTIRIN**
- **Manufacturer:** Wyeth
- **Use:** Pain relief
- **Dosage Form:** Tablet
- **Administration:** Oral
- **Ingredients:** Ethoheptazine citrate 75 mg (analgesic); aspirin 325 mg (analgesic/antipyretic).

ZACTIRIN is a fixed-combination product prescribed and promoted for the relief of mild to moderate pain. This mixture is comprised of ethoheptazine (Zactane), rated as lacking substantial evidence of effectiveness by the FDA, and aspirin, a proven pain-reliever. There is no evidence that the addition of ethoheptazine adds anything to the effectiveness of aspirin. For relief of mild to moderate pain, aspirin or acetaminophen (Tylenol) is recommended.

See similar drug ZACTIRIN COMPOUND-100, pg. 191

- **Brand Name:** ZACTIRIN COMPOUND-100
- **Manufacturer:** Wyeth
- **Use:** Pain relief
- **Dosage Form:** Tablet
- **Administration:** Oral
- **Ingredients:** Ethoheptazine citrate 100 mg, phenacetin 162 mg (analgesics); aspirin 227 mg (analgesic/antipyretic); caffeine 32 mg (stimulant).

ZACTIRIN COMPOUND-100 is a poly-

pharmaceutical prescribed and promoted for the relief of mild to moderate pain. Aside from a few trivial inclusions, this product is virtually the same as Zactirin. It contains ethoheptazine (Zactane), aspirin and phenacetin (proven pain-relievers), and caffeine. There are a number of products which contain APC (aspirin, phenacetin and caffeine), either alone or in combination with other ingredients, for pain-relief. However, aspirin alone is preferred. Phenacetin, when used on an extended basis, may have toxic effects on the kidneys and has been implicated as a carcinogen in man.

According to the *AMA Drug Evaluations* (second edition, pg. 272), the use of Zactirin and Zactirin Compound-100 is not recommended. It states that "in view of the equivocal analgesic effectiveness of ethoheptazine alone and the lack of evidence demonstrating that these mixtures provide an analgesic effect greater than aspirin alone, the rationale for their use is highly questionable."

The FDA has downgraded Zactirin Compound-100 to lacking substantial evidence of effectiveness as a fixed-combination.

For mild to moderate pain, aspirin or acetaminophen (if one is susceptible to stomach problems or allergic to aspirin) is the drug of choice. Phenacetin can cause kidney damage, kidney cancer and tumors of the nose and urinary tract.

See similar drug SYNALGOS, pg. 174, for discussion of APC.

Part IV:
HISTORY OF
INEFFECTIVE
PRESCRIPTION
DRUGS

1962 Drug Amendment and Review Procedures

In 1962, Congress amended the Food, Drug and Cosmetic Act of 1938 to require that all prescription drugs introduced after 1962 be proven effective before they could be marketed to the general public.* The 1962 amendment also applied to drugs approved for public use between 1938 and 1962. Knowledge of the existence of this important law might lead the consumer to believe that the drugs he or she takes today are of proven effectiveness. However, the 607 individual prescription drug products listed in this book that have been determined to lack evidence of effectiveness by the Food and Drug Administration are still on the market today—many of them the most widely prescribed medicines. Governmental inefficiency, lethargy and timidity, orchestrated by heavy

---

* Drugs introduced before 1938 were not bound by these new requirements of evidence of effectiveness as long as their manufacturers did not alter their composition, dosage form or labeling. In fact, there are very few drugs now available that still qualify for this "grandfather" exception.

pressure from drug companies to keep these drugs on the market, have permitted these products to continue to be prescribed to unsuspecting patients, sometimes by unsuspecting doctors.

In passing the 1962 drug law amendments, Congress wanted to clarify standards for assessing the effectiveness of drug claims. A drug manufacturer's declaration of effectiveness had to be supported by "substantial evidence," that is, "well-controlled investigations, including clinical evaluations, by experts qualified by scientific training and experience to evaluate the effectiveness of the drug involved. . . ." Congress gave the Secretary of the then Department of Health, Education and Welfare (HEW) the power to withdraw approval for a drug if "substantial evidence" of effectiveness was lacking. Prior to 1962, the drug industry had commonly relied on poorly controlled studies, clinical impressions and undocumented subjective opinions of physicians to support their promotional claims of effectiveness.

To review all prescription drugs approved for marketing between 1938 and 1962, the FDA entered into a contract with the National Academy of Sciences-National Research Council (NAS-NRC) in 1966. Drug manufacturers were asked to submit data to the NAS-NRC to support their claims of effectiveness and thirty panels of doctors, each composed of six experts in a particular field of drug therapy, were chosen to review the claims.

The NAS-NRC panels then placed each drug under one of the following classifications:

(1) *Effective:* The indication (i.e., use) meets the requirements of "substantial evidence" and the drug is effective.

(2) *Effective with Reservations:* The indication may meet the requirement if the composition of this product is changed or the labeling clarified.

(3) *Probably Effective:* The indication needs additional or supporting data or clarification.

(4) *Possibly Effective:* Substantial research is needed to substantiate the indications.*

(5) *Ineffective:* The indication lacks substantial evidence of effectiveness.

In early 1968, the FDA began to act on these NAS-NRC reports, the last of which was submitted in 1969. The entire review process lasted for over two years, with almost 4,000 drug formulations being examined. Each evaluation was to be completely assessed by the FDA and then

* According to one former NAS-NRC scientific panelist, "this designation means that in the best judgment of the panel members, if appropriate controlled studies were to be done, the result would be negative". . . . *(U.S. Medicine* February 15, 1971, pg. 26.)

released to the public by publishing it in the *Federal Register.**

After publicly announcing the classification of a drug, the early FDA policy gave the drug company a period of time (ranging from 30 days to 12 months, depending on the classification) in which to produce any additional substantial evidence of effectiveness. During this time, the drug companies were, as they are today, permitted to continue marketing these less-than-effective products. The FDA was supposed to begin withdrawal procedures if no substantial evidence of effectiveness was provided by the end of the interim period, but the FDA's efforts fell far short of this goal.

APHA Law Suit (1970) and Court Order (1972)

In 1970, as a challenge to the FDA's unwillingness to expedite the removal of less-than-effective drug products, the American Public Health Association (APHA) and the National Council of Senior Citizens filed a suit against the FDA challenging the legality of the manner in which that governmental agency was administering the new sections of the Act.

First, they charged that the FDA practice of giving drug manufacturers time to attempt to strengthen the record of a drug's effectiveness, after both the FDA and the independent scientific panels of the NAS-NRC had evaluated the drug (and found it deficient), violated federal law. Second, the plaintiffs claimed that the FDA often failed to follow up and carry out its own withdrawal guidelines.

Furthermore, the APHA charged that the FDA was responsible for excessive delays in scheduling drug company-requested hearings, thus further impeding the removal process. By 1970, less than half of the NAS-NRC reports had even been evaluated by the FDA and released to the public, let alone acted upon by that agency. This snail's pace did not bode well for the prospect of clearing the market of those drugs that had insufficient proof of clinical effectiveness.

The FDA's early pattern of inefficiency and lethargy in dealing with the task of withdrawing the ineffective drugs was only partially redressed by the Federal District Court's 1972 order in the APHA suit. Judge William Bryant concluded that there was no compelling reason why the remaining NAS-NRC drug evaluation reports should not immediately be released, and he explicitly directed the FDA to proceed as quickly as possible. The court also held that the 30-day to 12-month period for sub-

---

* The *Federal Register* is a daily compendium of all the public regulations and legal notices issued by Federal agencies.

mitting additional data was illegal, but constructed generous, yet specific, deadlines by which the FDA was required to complete its final effectiveness evaluations.

The 1972 Court Order seems to have been a mixed blessing. On the one hand, it criticized the FDA's apparent unwillingness and/or inability to resolve the situation promptly; it also served as a catalyst in forcing the rapid evaluation and release of all the remaining NAS-NRC reports. On the other hand, the deadlines established for issuing notices of opportunity for hearings on these less-than-effective drugs were extremely long, especially in light of the fact that manufacturers were free to market the drugs during this period. Even the most lenient timetables created by the Court Order expired in 1976; yet hundreds of less-than-effective drug products remain on the market today.

Paragraph XIV and "Exempt Drugs"

The 1972 Court Order contained a special paragraph (XIV) that stated that a "limited" number of drugs could remain on the market, pending the completion of scientific studies to determine their effectiveness, where there is a "compelling justification of the medical need for the drug." Ironically, although the 1962 drug law amendments were designed to eliminate the consideration of "marketplace opinion" from the process of drug marketing approval,* the Court's creation of the paragraph XIV loophole revitalized this element. Today, there are drug products with this protective status. They are temporarily "exempt" from the withdrawal procedures set up by the FDA for drugs that lack adequate evidence of effectiveness. Many of the so-called paragraph XIV drugs were cited as "ineffective" by the initial NAS-NRC scientific panels. However, because the FDA has seen fit to declare them of pressing medical need (How can there be a compelling need for ineffective drugs?) they are currently exempt. These particular drugs are supposedly inviolable so long as further studies are being conducted to clarify their efficacy status. However, appropriate studies for many of the different drug groups comprising the "exempt" products have never been conducted, while some were completed over three years ago.**

There is no consistently applied standard for deciding which drugs are of compelling medical need and therefore merit temporary exemption. The reasons vary considerably and usually contradict the spirit of the

---

* Approval was to be based solely on "substantial evidence" of safety and effectiveness.
** Answers to interrogatories submitted by the FDA to William Schultz, Public Citizen Attorney, April 16, 1979, in the recently revitalized *APHA v. Harris* suit.

1962 Drug Act and the 1972 Court Order. The FDA often justifies the exemption of certain ineffective drug groups because of a perception that physicians rely heavily on these products and are convinced of their usefulness.

The number of these medicines used in serious medical conditions with no effective alternatives available is small. However, rather than including only a "limited" number of potentially valuable drugs, with as yet unproven effectiveness, the FDA has exempted large numbers of prescription medicines that should have been removed from the market long ago.

In general, when the FDA announces publicly that a certain drug or class of drugs is being placed in the paragraph XIV "exempt" category, no clarification is provided as to the duration of the additional tests to be conducted and why the drug is thought to be needed by the medical community. In fact, the FDA has never formally informed the medical profession or the public of the scientific status of these drug products.

Most of the paragraph XIV drugs have been "exempt" since 1972 and, according to the FDA's own estimations, final decisions regarding effectiveness for the bulk of them won't be reached until 1981 or later. In the meantime, physicians unknowingly continue to prescribe, and consumers continue to use, these "exempt" drugs that have not been shown to be clinically effective.

At present, many less-than-effective drug products have not been placed under temporary "exemption." These products are the clearest example of the FDA's blatant non-compliance with the 1972 Court Order,* since the last deadline for withdrawal expired October 1976. With respect to these one hundred-odd drugs, the FDA has either failed to (1) initiate the procedures necessary to hold a hearing for the drug company on the question of withdrawing market approval, or (2) respond to a company request for such a hearing. As one top FDA official put it, "the FDA has not acted quickly because it hasn't been under pressure to do so."

According to a federal Manpower Management Study performed in October-November 1978, less than 5 percent of the working time of the average professional reviewer in the FDA's Bureau of Drugs is spent implementing the Drug Effectiveness project. Given the extremely limited commitment by the FDA to the task of removing these old

---

*The subject of renewed litigation by Public Citizen attorneys representing the APHA and the National Council of Senior Citizens. A settlement was reached in this litigation in September, 1980 with FDA agreeing to do the following: 1) add more staff to expedite the project 2) give priority to the biggest selling drugs 3) notify all doctors of the names of all drugs which lack evidence of effectiveness, including those which FDA has "exempted" from removal.

prescription drugs of unproven effectiveness, it is easy to see why so many of these products remain on the market today. FDA lethargy stems from a combination of entangling regulatory procedures, inefficiency, lack of commitment of adequate resources and a reluctance to use the courts to remove these drugs. Drug manufacturers still earn large sums of money from the sale of ineffective drugs. Their threat of protracted legal battles has, thus far, successfully cowed FDA attempts to withdraw most of the big-selling ineffective drugs.

In addition to the drug products which are part of the primary FDA Drug Efficacy project, three other groups of ineffective drugs are included in this book.

The papaverine/ethaverine drugs (67 products) in this book are blood-vessel dilating drugs which are promoted for the treatment of poor blood circulation of the head, limbs or heart. Because of yet undetermined factors, these drugs were never reviewed as part of the primary Drug Efficacy project, but more recently have been found by both the FDA and an FDA Advisory Committee to lack evidence of effectiveness and safety. (See more detailed discussion of these drugs on pg. 27).

There are also numerous drugs used for treating vaginal infections which are called *vaginal sulfonamides.* These also were not part of the primary Drug Efficacy Project but have been found by an FDA Advisory Committee to lack evidence of effectiveness. (See pg. 53 for a more detailed discussion of these drugs.)

The third group is neomycin-containing drugs used for direct application to the skin, which an FDA Advisory Committee on over-the-counter drugs has concluded lack evidence of effectiveness. (See Part II: Drugs for Skin, Eye or Ear for a more detailed discussion of these drugs.)

APPENDIX A

1979 TOTAL

Drug	1979 Total Rx Filled	Estimated 1979 Retail Sales
Achrostatin-V	280,000	$ 2,800,000
Actifed	12,900,000	49,000,000
Actifed-C Expectorant	2,700,000	12,700,000
Adrenosem Salicylate	40,000	330,000
Adroyd	6,000	60,000
Aerosporin Otic Solution	50,000	100,000
Alevaire	6,000	30,000
Ambenyl Expectorant	1,800,000	9,800,000
Amesec	290,000	2,000,000
Aminobrain P-T	No Data	No Data
Aminophylline and Amytal	No Data	No Data
Amodrine	40,000	250,000
Ananase-50,-100	440,000	3,300,000
Antora-B T.D.	3,000	30,000
Arlidin	1,100,000	11,900,000
Asminyl	No Data	No Data
Ataraxoid	210,000	1,800,000
Avazyme	30,000	310,000
AVC Cream	1,600,000	12,000,000
AVC/Dienestrol Cream	270,000	2,300,000
AVC Suppositories	620,000	5,000,000
Azo-Gantanol	940,000	7,200,000
Azotrex	120,000	1,700,000
Bacimycin	10,000	20,000
Barbidonna	120,000	610,000
Belladenal	120,000	780,000
Benadryl with Ephedrine	10,000	90,000
Bentyl	2,500,000	15,500,000
Bentyl with Phenobarbital	1,200,000	8,200,000
Benylin Cough Syrup	2,300,000	8,900,000
Berocca-C	20,000	80,000
Berocca-C 500	No Data	No Data

Drug	1979 Total Rx Filled	Estimated 1979 Retail Sales
Betadine Vaginal Gel	270,000	$ 2,500,000
Biozyme Ointment	100,000	No Data
Blephamide Liquifilm	390,000	2,100,000
Butazolidin Alka	5,700,000	34,800,000
Butibel	370,000	1,400,000
Butigetic	50,000	280,000
Butiserpazide Prestabs 25, 50	110,000	600,000
Caldecort	30,000	220,000
Cantil with Phenobarbital	180,000	1,700,000
Carbrital Kapseals	320,000	2,000,000
Carbrital Kapseals Half Strength	10,000	60,000
Cardilate	500,000	3,400,000
Cardilate-P	No Data	No Data
Cartrax 10, 20	20,000	230,000
Cenalene	9,000	70,000
Cetacaine	No Data	No Data
Chardonna-2	170,000	780,000
Chloromycetin-HC	200,000	1,100,000
Chlorpheniramine Maleate	No Data	No Data
Chymoral	290,000	3,500,000
Circubid	No Data	No Data
Clistin Expectorant	60,000	230,000
Clistin R-A	50,000	370,000
Combid Spansules	2,700,000	22,000,000
Co-Pyronil	640,000	4,900,000
Co-Pyronil Pediatric	60,000	400,000
Cordran-N	230,000	1,900,000
Cor-Tar-Quin	120,000	900,000
Cortisporin Cream	130,000	570,000
Cortisporin Ointment	400,000	2,700,000
Cortisporin Ophthalmic	780,000	4,100,000
Cyclospasmol	1,400,000	15,700,000
Dainite	No Data	No Data
Dainite-KI	20,000	110,000
Daricon PB	30,000	220,000
Deaner	30,000	260,000

Drug	1979 Total Rx Filled	Estimated 1979 Retail Sales
Deca-Durabolin	6,000	$ 120,000
Decaspray	250,000	1,600,000
Declostatin	70,000	1,000,000
Declostatin-300	40,000	430,000
Deprol	330,000	4,600,000
Dexamyl	400,000	2,300,000
Dianabol	150,000	1,600,000
Dimetane Expectorant	2,000,000	8,700,000
Dimetane Expectorant-DC	1,600,000	8,500,000
Dimetapp Elixir	7,900,000	32,000,000
Dimetapp Extentabs	6,900,000	35,000,000
Disophrol	690,000	4,400,000
Diutensen	240,000	2,800,000
Donnatal	8,400,000	29,000,000
Donnatal Extentabs	570,000	2,700,000
Donphen	No Data	No Data
Duotrate Plateau Caps	40,000	440,000
D-Vaso	30,000	260,000
Enarax 5, 10	30,000	500,000
Equagesic	2,900,000	21,100,000
Esgic	140,000	840,000
Eskatrol Spansules	810,000	6,300,000
Ethatab	190,000	2,000,000
F-E-P Creame	130,000	880,000
Folbesyn	2,000	60,000
Forhistal Lontabs	40,000	270,000
Gevizol	No Data	No Data
Hybephen	30,000	110,000
Hycodan	1,100,000	5,500,000
Hydrocortisone-Neomycin	No Data	No Data
Ilotycin Topical	120,000	No Data
Indogesic	No Data	No Data
Isordil Sublingual	2,100,000	16,200,000
Isordil Tembids	1,100,000	11,600,000
Isordil Titradose & Chewable Tablets	3,900,000	33,600,000
Isordil with Phenobarbital	70,000	630,000

Drug	1979 Total Rx Filled	Estimated 1979 Retail Sales
Isovex-100	20,000	$ 200,000
Kinesed	460,000	2,200,000
Lapav	No Data	No Data
Levsin w/Phenobarbital	100,000	740,000
Librax	5,600,000	46,000,000
Lidosporin Otic	600,000	No Data
Luftodil	No Data	No Data
Lufyllin-EPG	10,000	110,000
Mannitol Hexanitrate	No Data	No Data
Mannitol Hexanitrate w/Phenobarbital	No Data	No Data
Marax & Marax DF	2,100,000	13,900,000
Marplan	60,000	500,000
Medrol Enpak	No Data	No Data
Mepergan Fortis	390,000	2,200,000
Metimyd	250,000	1,600,000
Metrazol	40,000	270,000
Migral	20,000	170,000
Miltrate	40,000	670,000
M.V.I. Injection	2,000	10,000
Mycolog	6,300,000	51,000,000
Mysteclin F	1,100,000	10,500,000
Naturetin with K	210,000	1,800,000
Neo-Cort-Dome	60,000	290,000
Neo-Cortef Ophthalmic	90,000	520,000
Neo-Cortef Topical	110,000	900,000
Neo-Decadron Ophthalmic	840,000	4,700,000
Neo-Decadron Topical	150,000	870,000
Neo-Delta-Cortef Ophthalmic	60,000	330,000
Neo-Delta-Cortef-Topical	No Data	No Data
Neo-Hydeltrasol Ophthalmic	20,000	100,000
Neo-Medrol Acetate	90,000	770,000
Neo-Medrol Ophthalmic	20,000	70,000
Neo-Oxylone	3,000	10,000
Neopavrin Forte	4,000	60,000
Neosone	No Data	No Data
Neosporin	890,000	No Data
Neosporin-G	460,000	No Data
Neo-Synalar	270,000	2,000,000

Drug	1979 Total Rx Filled	Estimated 1979 Retail Sales
Nico-Metrazol	30,000	$ 310,000
Nitro-Bid Ointment	490,000	3,600,000
Nitro-Bid Plateau Caps	2,600,000	22,800,000
Nitroglyn	50,000	380,000
Numorphan Rectal Suppositories	10,000	150,000
Nystaform-HC	20,000	130,000
Omni-Tuss	60,000	370,000
Ophthocort	90,000	640,000
Orenzyme	190,000	2,800,000
Ornade Spansules	4,800,000	27,000,000
Orthoxine Hydrochloride	20,000	180,000
Otobiotic	210,000	No Data
Otocort	10,000	60,000
Oxaine M	410,000	2,100,000
Oxsoralen	30,000	410,000
Papase	150,000	1,000,000
Papavatral LA w/Phenobarbital	9,000	90,000
Papaverine	960,000	5,500,000
Parafon Forte	3,800,000	28,400,000
Parnate	220,000	1,500,000
Pathibamate	880,000	9,900,000
Pathilon w/Phenobarbital	30,000	280,000
Pathilon Sequels	10,000	100,000
Pavabid HP	50,000	630,000
Pavabid Plateau	3,300,000	31,300,000
Pavakey-300	7,000	70,000
Paveril Phosphate	20,000	100,000
PBZ w/Ephedrine	30,000	150,000
PBZ Expectorant w/Ephedrine	110,000	440,000
PBZ Expectorant w/Ephedrine & Codeine	100,000	450,000
PBZ Lontabs & PBZ-SR	280,000	1,800,000
Pentritol	10,000	200,000
Pentryate Stronger	No Data	No Data
Peritrate	770,000	6,000,000

Drug	1979 Total Rx Filled	Estimated 1979 Retail Sales
Peritrate w/Phenobarbital	150,000	$ 1,100,000
Persantine	3,600,000	53,000,000
Phenergan Expectorant w/Codeine	4,000,000	19,500,000
Phenergan Expectorant Pediatric w/Dextromethorphan	890,000	3,900,000
Phenergan Expectorant Plain	2,400,000	9,900,000
Phenergan VC Expectorant w/Codeine	2,900,000	15,200,000
Phenergan VC Expectorant Plain	1,700,000	7,700,000
Phenobarbital w/Atropine	No Data	No Data
Potaba	40,000	360,000
Priscoline	70,000	520,000
Priscoline Lontabs	4,000	50,000
Pro-Banthine w/Dartal	80,000	1,000,000
Pro-Banthine w/Phenobarbital	250,000	2,400,000
Propion Vaginal Gel	30,000	200,000
Proternol	No Data	No Data
Quadrinal	400,000	3,000,000
Quibron Plus	190,000	1,400,000
Rautrax	30,000	540,000
Rautrax-N	110,000	2,200,000
Rautrax-N Modified	10,000	200,000
Repan	50,000	280,000
Robinul-PH	70,000	410,000
Robinul-PH Forte	9,000	60,000
Roniacol	110,000	1,300,000
Roniacol Timespan Tabs	430,000	5,000,000
Ru-Vert	730,000	5,100,000
Sidonna	20,000	90,000
Spectrocin	3,000	10,000
Spentane T.D.	No Data	No Data
Sulfathalidine	100,000	590,000
Synalgos	220,000	1,000,000
Synalgos-DC	3,100,000	16,100,000
Tarcortin	No Data	No Data
Teldrin	1,500,000	7,800,000
Terra-Cortril Ophthalmic	80,000	350,000
Terra-Cortril Topical	120,000	580,000

Drug	1979 Total Rx Filled	Estimated 1979 Retail Sales
Terrastatin	110,000	$ 1,100,000
Therapav	20,000	210,000
Tigan Rectal Suppositories	1,000,000	5,400,000
Trocinate	50,000	380,000
Tussionex	1,400,000	9,000,000
Tuss-Ornade	3,000,000	16,400,000
Urobiotic-250	250,000	3,700,000
Valpin 50-PB	140,000	1,100,000
Vasocon-A	810,000	4,700,000
Vasodilan	2,100,000	29,000,000
Vioform-Hydrocortisone	1,300,000	9,800,000
Vioform-Hydrocortisone Mild	380,000	2,200,000
Vita-Metrazol	50,000	410,000
Vytone	190,000	1,100,000
Winstrol	80,000	850,000
Wyanoids HC Rectal Suppositories	550,000	4,700,000
Zactane	No Data	No Data
Zactirin	110,000	710,000
Zactirin Compound-100	200,000	1,400,000

APPENDIX B

1979 TOP 30 LESS-THAN-EFFECTIVE PRESCRIPTION DRUGS*
(All Among Top 200 Drugs in U.S.)

Rank	Product	Firm	# Rx[1]	Retail[1] Sales
1	Dimetapp (2)	Robins	14,800,000	$67,000,000
2	Actifed	Burroughs Wellcome	12,900,000	49,000,000
3	Donnatal (2)	Robins	9,000,000	31,700,000
4	Isordil (3)	Ives	7,100,000	61,400,000
5	Mycolog	Squibb	6,300,000	51,000,000
6	Butazolidin Alka	Geigy	5,700,000	34,800,000
7	Librax	Roche	5,600,000	46,000,000
8	Ornade Spansules	Smith Kline & French	4,800,000	27,000,000
9	Phenergan Expectorant w/Codeine	Wyeth	4,000,000	19,500,000
10	Parafon Forte	McNeil	3,800,000	28,400,000
11	Persantine	Boehringer-Ingelheim	3,600,000	53,000,000
12	Pavabid Plateau	Marion	3,300,000	31,300,000
13	Synalgos-DC	Ives	3,100,000	16,100,000
14	Tuss-Ornade	Smith Kline & French	3,000,000	16,400,000
15	Phenergan VC Expectorant w/Codeine	Wyeth	2,900,000	15,200,000
	Equagesic	Wyeth	2,900,000	21,100,000
17	Actifed-C Expectorant	Burroughs Wellcome	2,700,000	12,700,000
	Combid Spansules	Smith Kline & French	2,700,000	22,000,000
19	Nitro-Bid Plateau Caps	Marion	2,600,000	22,800,000
20	Bentyl	Merrell-National	2,500,000	15,500,000
21	Phenergan Expectorant Plain	Wyeth	2,400,000	9,900,000
22	Benylin Cough Syrup	Parke-Davis	2,300,000	8,900,000
23	Marax and Marax DF	Roerig	2,100,000	13,900,000
	Vasodilan	Mead Johnson	2,100,000	29,000,000
25	Dimetane Expectorant	Robins	2,000,000	8,700,000
26	Ambenyl Expectorant	Marion	1,800,000	9,800,000
27	Phenergan VC Expectorant Plain	Wyeth	1,700,000	7,700,000
28	Dimetane Expectorant-DC	Robins	1,600,000	8,500,000
	AVC Cream	Merrell-National	1,600,000	12,000,000
30	Teldrin	Smith Kline & French	1,500,000	7,800,000

[1]1979 National Prescription Audit, IMS America Ltd., Ambler, PA.

*Based on prescriptions filled.

APPENDIX C
HOW THIS BOOK WAS COMPILED

Lack of Effectiveness

Most of the entries in this book were part of the original National Academy of Sciences-National Research Council (NAS-NRC) review of the effectiveness of prescription drugs. These drugs appear in the *FDA Interim Trade Name Index of All Prescription Drugs in the Drug Efficacy Study-Cumulative up to August 1, 1980* or are identical or related to drugs appearing in this Index. These drugs are either rated "ineffective" by the FDA or, though lacking substantial evidence of effectiveness, are exempt under the paragraph XIV provisions (See History pg. 196). Other drug entries, while not officially part of the original Drug Efficacy Study, have been subsequently reviewed by the NAS-NRC and their labeling information and/or entry in the 1980 *Physicians' Desk Reference* contains a box stating that they have been found to be less-than-effective. The remaining entries have been reviewed by the FDA either individually or as a class, have been found to lack evidence of effectiveness and have been announced as such in the Federal Register (papaverines and ethaverines) or by FDA Advisory Committees (vaginal sulfonamides and topical antibiotics).

The identical drugs in the index (i.e. those which refer the reader directly to another drug) are the same as the entry referred to in active ingredients, strength and dosage form. These identical drugs are either from one of the above mentioned sources or were gathered from the FDA's computer printout *Report Number DRLS-360 Ingredient List by Firm* (April 29, 1980) which lists drugs by ingredients or from *Facts and Comparisons* (August 1980).

Availability

The drugs in this book are all available from most large pharmacies. All of these drugs are listed in *Facts and Comparisons* (August 1980). A small number of the drugs are no longer being produced by their manufacturers; however, a telephone survey of Washington, D.C. area pharmacies in July 1980 showed these drugs to still be readily available.

Sales and Rx Data

Sales data are from the *National Prescription Audit: Therapeutic Category Report* (IMS America, Ltd, Ambler, PA, 1979).

GLOSSARY

ADRENAL CORTICOSTEROIDS: Drugs identical or similar to those produced by the adrenal gland which act as anti-inflammatory agents or control the body's salt/water balance.

ADRENERGIC: Of or relating to the type of chemical activity characteristic of epinephrine and similar substances. These drugs and bodily substances are often called the sympathomimetics, because they activate organs and blood vessels via the sympathetic ("fight-flight") branch of the autonomic (involuntary) nervous system.

ALLERGY: A response of the body's immune system in certain people upon exposure to a drug, food, or other substance. The reaction is mediated by a special type of antibody (IgE) as well as certain chemicals, such as histamine. The response can vary tremendously, from a simple rash (hives) to death (anaphylactic shock).

ALZHEIMER'S DISEASE: (Presenile dementia). A form of degenerative, organic brain disease, often affecting the entire frontal and temporal lobes of the brain cortex (sites of memory, learning, etc).

ANABOLIC: An agent that promotes the conversion of a simple substance into more complex compounds; a "building up" of cells and tissues.

ANALEPTIC: A central nervous system stimulant used to maintain vital functions during severe central nervous system depression.

ANALGESIC: Pain reliever.

ANAPHYLAXIS: Extreme life-threatening allergic reaction.

ANDROGEN: A drug or hormone that promotes the development and maintenance of the male sex characteristics and structure.

ANEMIA: Decrease in red blood cells or in hemoglobin in the blood.

ANESTHETIC: A drug that produces local or general loss of sensation.

ANGINA PECTORIS: Chest pain due to coronary artery disease, often extending into the neck and arms. Episodes are relieved by rest or prevented by nitroglycerin taken under the tongue (sublingually).

ANKYLOSING SPONDYLITIS: See Rheumatoid Spondylitis.

ANTACID: Agents used to neutralize excess stomach acid. Often used in ulcer therapy.

ANTI-ANXIETY: A drug used to treat the symptoms of anxiety, e.g. fear, restlessness, nervous tension.

ANTIASTHMATIC: A drug used to treat the symptoms of asthma and related respiratory conditions, including shortness of breath and wheezing. These drugs usually dilate breathing passages.

ANTIBACTERIAL: A substance which kills or prevents the growth of bacteria. Most antibacterial drugs have a limited spectrum of activity and therefore are effective for only particular bacteria.

ANTIBIOTIC: A drug derived from molds or bacteria which impedes or eliminates the growth of other bacteria or fungi.

ANTICHOLINERGIC: A drug that blocks the effects of acetylcholine, a chemical which is produced naturally by the body and is responsible for certain nervous system activities (parasympathetic). Anticholinergic drugs inhibit the secretion of acid in the stomach, slow the passage of food through the digestive system, inhibit the production of saliva, sweat, and bronchial secretions, and increase the heart rate.

ANTICOAGULANT: A drug which inhibits or slows blood clotting.

ANTI-DEPRESSANT: A drug used to treat the symptoms of depression.

ANTIDIARRHEAL: A drug used to treat diarrhea.

ANTIFUNGAL: An antibiotic that kills or inhibits fungi.

ANTIHISTAMINE: A drug used to lessen or counteract the effects of histamine, a chemical produced by the body in response to various allergy-causing agents. It is used in many products to relieve the symptoms of allergy. Many antihistamines have undesirable side effects, such as drowsiness, and should be used with caution.

ANTIHYPERTENSIVE: A drug that lowers blood pressure.

ANTIINFECTIVE: A drug used to combat infection by killing disease-causing microorganisms.

ANTI-INFLAMMATORY: A drug used to reduce inflammation, a reaction of tissues to injury.

ANTINAUSEANT: A drug that suppresses nausea, especially that due to motion sickness.

ANTIPRURITIC: A drug used to relieve itching.

ANTIPYRETIC: A drug used to reduce fever.

ANTISEPTIC: A substance that inhibits the growth and development of microorganisms without necessarily destroying them.

ANTISPASMODIC: A drug agent used to quiet the spasms of voluntary and involuntary muscles, usually of the gastrointestinal tract (stomach and intestines).

ANTITUSSIVE: A drug used to suppress cough. Can be narcotic (e.g. codeine) or non-narcotic (e.g. dextromethorphan).

ANXIETY: A feeling of apprehension, uncertainty and fear.

ARTERIOSCLEROSIS: Changes in arteries consisting of thickening of the walls, loss of elasticity and sometimes calcium deposition; "hardening of the arteries."

ARTERY: A vessel carrying oxygenated blood from the heart to the tissues.

ARTHRITIS: An inflammation and swelling or stiffness of a joint.

ATHEROSCLEROSIS: Changes in arteries consisting of build-up of cholesterol and other substances, resulting in decrease of flow through particular arteries.

ATROPHY: A wasting away; degenerative process.

BRONCHITIS: An inflammation of the bronchi (air passages of the lung).

BRONCHODILATOR: Drug which acts to widen the lung's air passages (bronchi). There are several classes of these drugs which differ in both chemical composition and pharmacological properties. Some bronchodilators (e.g. theophylline) dilate the airways directly by relaxing the smooth muscle walls. Others (e.g. ephedrine) interact with sympathetic nervous system activities to relax the smooth muscle walls.

BRONCHOSPASM: Temporary narrowing of the major breathing passageways due to violent, involuntary contraction of the smooth muscle walls. Results in asthma-like symptoms.

CARCINOMA: A malignant, cancerous growth.

CARDIAC: Relating to the heart.

CEREBRAL: Relating to the brain.

CEREBRUM: That part of the brain which controls the conscious mental processes and is the seat of memory.

CONGESTION: An abnormal accumulation of blood or tissue fluid in the vessels of an organism.

CORONARY ARTERY: Blood vessel that supplies the heart tissue.

CORTICOSTEROID: See Adrenal Corticosteroid. A hormone of the adrenal cortex, or a synthetic analog.

CUTANEOUS: Pertaining to the skin.

DECONGESTANT: A drug that reduces congestion.

DEMENTIA: Deterioration or loss of intellectual faculties, reasoning power, will, and memory due to organic brain disease; characterized by confusion, disorientation, and stupor of varying degrees.

DERMATITIS: An inflammation of the skin.

DILATE: To enlarge (a cavity, blood vessel, or opening).

DISINFECTANT: An agent that destroys disease-causing microorganisms on contact.

DIURETIC: A drug that increases the volume of urine.

DIVERTICULITIS: Inflammation of an outpouching of the intestine.

DOSE: Quantity of a drug or medicine to be taken or applied.

DRUG: A substance used as a medicine.

DRUG INTERACTION: Case where one drug affects (increases or decreases) the therapeutic or toxic effects of a second drug. This can present serious problems with patients taking more than one drug. (Remember that alcohol is a drug which can interact with many other drugs).

DYSMENORRHEA: Painful menstruation.

ECZEMA: An inflammatory disease of the skin characterized by redness, swelling, blistering, watery discharge, scales and crust.

EDEMA: Build-up of watery fluid in the tissues of the body; also known as "water weight."

ELECTROLYTES: Important chemicals, such as sodium, potassium, calcium and bicarbonate, found in the body tissues and fluids.

EMBOLISM: Occlusion of a blood vessel by a blood clot or a large mass of foreign material. Causes various syndromes depending on the size of the vessel obstructed, the organ and tissue it supplies, and the nature of the mass.

ENZYME: A special protein made by the body cells which greatly speeds up a particular chemical reaction in the body. Enzymes are highly specific catalysts which remain unchanged during the reaction.

ESTROGEN: A drug or hormone that has activity on female sex organs or maintains female sex characteristics.

EXFOLIATION: A peeling and shedding of the superficial layer of the skin or other tissue.

EXPECTORANT: A drug that is supposed to stimulate the production of secretions from mucous membranes (e.g. bronchi) and "thin" these secretions. Used in a number of cold remedies to loosen phlegm so that it can be coughed up.

FDA: Food and Drug Administration.

FEVER: Body temperature above normal (98.6°F/37°C).

GASTRITIS: Inflammation of the stomach.

GENERIC: Standard name accepted for a drug. Non-proprietary, i.e. not protected by a trademark.

HEART BLOCK: Failure of the conduction tissue of the heart to conduct impulses normally from one part of the heart to another, causing altered rhythm of the heartbeat. There are varying degrees of severity. Slow heartbeat with fainting, seizure or even death, results from this abnormality.

HEPATITIS: An inflammation of the liver.

HISTAMINE: A chemical made by the body especially during an allergic reaction; it produces dilation of small blood vessels, lowers the blood pressure, and increases secretions from the stomach, the salivary glands, and other organs.

HRG: Health Research Group (Washington, D.C.).

HYPEREMIA: Increased blood in a section of the body; may be active, when due to dilation of vessels, or passive, when drainage is hindered.

HYPERKALEMIA: Abnormally high levels of potassium in the blood.

HYPERMOTILITY: Increased movement of food and gastrointestinal contents through the stomach and intestines, often associated with muscle spasm and pain. Rapid clearing of the stomach often aggravates stomach ulcer and intensifies pain.

HYPERTENSION: High blood pressure.

HYPNOTIC: An agent that dulls the senses or induces sleep.

HYPOKALEMIA: Low levels of potassium in the blood.

HYPOTENSION: Low blood pressure.

INFLAMMATION: The succession of changes which occur in living tissue when it is injured, characterized by pain, redness and swelling.

INTERMITTENT CLAUDICATION: Cramp-like pains and weakness in the legs resulting from inadequate blood supply.

MALAISE: A general feeling of illness.

MIGRAINE HEADACHE: Pain on one side of the head; a recurrent, intense vascular headache, varying in intensity, frequency, and duration. Migraines are often associated with nausea and vomiting, and sensitivity to bright light.

NARCOTIC: A drug that produces insensibility or stupor, and relieves pain; a class of drug regulated by law.

NAS-NRC: National Academy of Sciences-National Research Council.

NCI: National Cancer Institute.

NOH: Notice of Opportunity for Hearing—The Food and Drug Administration's procedure for informing a drug manufacturer that its product lacks substantial evidence of effectiveness. When the FDA issues an NOH, it gives the manufacturer a chance to participate in a formal hearing to resolve FDA's proposal to withdraw the product from the market.

OBESITY: An increase of body weight due to the accumulation of fat, 10-20 percent beyond the normal range for a particular age, sex, and height.

OPHTHALMIC: Relating to the eye.

ORAL: Relating to the mouth.

OSTEOARTHRITIS: A special degenerative joint disease.

OTIC: Relating to the ear.

OTITIS: Inflammation of the ear.

OVER-THE-COUNTER DRUG: Medication sold without a prescription.

PARASYMPATHETIC NERVOUS SYSTEM: A division of the autonomic nervous system which helps to regulate a number of organ systems, such as the gastrointestinal, cardiovascular, and urinary systems and the muscles. It generally acts in opposition to the sympathetic nervous system.

PARENTERAL: Outside the intestine. Refers to a route of drug administration: under the skin, intravenous or intramuscular.

PARKINSONISM: A neurological disorder marked by tremor, muscular rigidity, and decreased muscular movement.

PDR: *Physicians' Desk Reference,* a semi-authoritative compendium of brand name prescription drugs published annually by Medical Economics, Inc.

PEPTIC ULCER: A localized loss of tissue, involving mainly the lining of areas of the digestive tract exposed to acid produced by the stomach. Usually involves the lower esophagus, the stomach, or the beginning of the small intestine.

PERIPHERAL ARTERIAL DISEASE: See Arteriosclerosis. The obstruction of peripheral arteries, such as those in the limbs. This results in a number of conditions, such as intermittent claudication.

PHLEBITIS: An inflammation of a vein.

PRESCRIPTION: Written formula for the preparation and administration of medicine, by a qualified, licensed medical doctor. Today it is a set of instructions for the pharmacist who dispenses the drug and the patient who consumes it.

PROPHYLACTIC: Tending to prevent disease.

PROTEOLYTIC ENZYME: An enzyme used to digest fibrous protein.

PSORIASIS: An inflammatory skin disease characterized by itching and scaling.

PRURITIS: Itching.

PSYCHOTHERAPEUTIC DRUG: Drug used as treatment or part of the treatment of emotional disorders. These disorders may or may not have a physical basis.

PULMONARY: Pertaining to the lungs.

PYODERMA: Any skin discharge characterized by pus formation.

RAYNAUD'S DISEASE: Intermittent paleness, redness, and coldness of the fingers and toes. The disease is rare in males.

RHEUMATOID SPONDYLITIS: Chronic, progressive disease involving the joints; may give rise to a stiff back. Occurs more frequently in women than men.

RHINITIS: Inflammation of the nasal passageways.

SEDATIVE: Any drug which produces a quieting or calming effect, relief.

SENSITIZE: To make susceptible to a specific substance.

SENILE DEMENTIA: A chronic organic brain syndrome associated with old age, usually characterized by difficulties in learning and organizing new information, childish behavior, self-centeredness, and general mental deterioration. May be caused by different disease states.

SKELETAL MUSCLE RELAXANT: A drug that inhibits contraction of voluntary muscles.

SUBLINGUAL: Administration of a drug under the tongue.

SUPPOSITORY: A solid medication introduced into different orifices of the body, e.g. anus, vagina.

STOKES-ADAMS: Fainting or seizure due to complete heart block.

SUPPRESSANT: A drug useful in the control, rather than the cure, of a disease.

SURFACTANT: An agent that decreases surface tension. Usually referring to the respiratory passages.

SYMPATHETIC NERVOUS SYSTEM: That part of the autonomic nervous system responsible for stimulating the body and preparing it for "fight or flight". It acts in opposition to the parasympathetic system in the regulation of organ systems. Epinephrine is one of the key mediators of the sympathetic system.

SYMPATHOMIMETIC: Drug with sympathetic action; effects include increased blood pressure and rapid heartbeat. Also causes relief of congestion by constricting blood vessels.

SYMPTOM: Any change in function, appearance, or sensation related to a disease.

TACHYCARDIA: Rapid heart rate.

TESTOSTERONE: Male sex hormone, an androgen.

TOPICAL: Local, external application of a drug to a particular place, usually the skin.

TOXIC: Poisonous or harmful.

TRANQUILIZER: A drug which acts to reduce mental tension and anxiety.

TRICHOMONIASIS: An infestation with parasitic protozoa of the genus Trichomonas.

ULCER: Localized loss of surface tissue of the skin or mucous membrane.

VAGINITIS: Inflammation of the vagina.

VASCULAR: Of or pertaining to blood vessels.

VASOCONSTRICTOR: A drug which constricts blood vessels, commonly used for nasal congestion.

VASODILATOR: Drug that causes opening or widening of blood vessels. Coronary vasodilator drugs have this effect on the coronary arteries in the heart.

VASOSPASM: Constriction of the blood vessels, due to a disease (e.g. Raynaud's disease), a disorder or drug (e.g. sympathomimetic).

VERTIGO: Sensation that the outside world is revolving about the patient or that he himself is spinning; dizziness, giddiness.

VESTIBULAR SYSTEM: The anatomical apparatus involved with the balance and orientation of the body.

VITAMIN: Chemical present in foods in small amounts that is essential to normal body functions. As a rule man is unable to synthesize these chemicals. They are effective in very small amounts and do not furnish energy, but are very important for the transformation of energy and for the regulation of metabolism.

BIBLIOGRAPHY

Abramowicz, Mark, ed., *The Medical Letter on Drugs and Therapeutics*, New Rochelle: The Medical Letter Inc., 1971.

American Medical Association Council on Drugs, *AMA Drug Evaluations*, first edition, Chicago: American Medical Association, 1971.

American Medical Association Department of Drugs, *AMA Drug Evaluations*, third edition, Littleton, MA: Publishing Sciences Group, 1977.

————————, *AMA Drug Evaluations*, second edition, Acton, MA: Publishing Sciences Group, 1973.

Armstrong, B. et al., "Retrospective study of the association between use of rauwolfia derivatives and breast cancer in English women," *Lancet* 2(7882):672-675, 1974.

Baker, C.E., ed., *Physicians' Desk Reference*, Oradell, NJ: Litton, 1980.

Besdine, R., "Treatable dementia in the elderly," presented at NIH Consensus Development Conference on Treatable Brain Diseases in the Elderly, Bethesda, MD, July 1978.

Billups, N.F. and S.M. Billups, eds., *American Drug Index*, Philadelphia: J. B. Lippincott, 1979.

Boston Collaborative Drug Surveillance Program, "Reserpine and breast cancer," *Lancet* 2(7882):669-671, 1974.

Burack, R. and F.J. Fox, *The New Handbook of Prescription Drugs*, revised edition, New York: Ballantine Books, 1975.

Coffman, J.D., "Vasodilator drugs in peripheral vascular disease," *New England J. Med.*, 300: 713-717, 1979.

Competitive Problems in the Drug Industry: Hearing Before the Subcommittee on Monopoly [Senate] Select Committee on Small Business, 33 vols., Washington: GPO, 1967-1977.

Davidov, M.E. and W.J. Mroczek, "The effect of nitroglycerin ointment on the exercise capacity of patients with angina pectoris," *Angiology*, 27:205-11, 1976.

Davies, D.M., ed., *Textbook of Adverse Drug Reactions*, Oxford: Oxford University Press, 1977.

Davis, C.M. et al., "The value of neomycin in a neomycin-steroid cream," *JAMA*, 203:298-300, 1968.

Epstein, E., "Allergy to dermatologic agents," *JAMA*, 198:517-520, 1966.

Food and Drug Administration, *FDA Drug Bulletin,* November 1979.

—————————, *Report Number DRLS-360 Ingredient List by Firm,* Drug Listing System, April 30, 1980.

—————————, *FD.1 Interim Trade Name Index of All Prescription Drugs in the Drug Efficacy Study-Cumulative up to August 1, 1980.*

Geffner, E.S., ed., *Compendium of Drug Therapy,* New York: Biomedical Information Corporation, 1980.

Goodman, L.S., and A. Gilman, *The Pharmacological Basis of Therapeutics,* fifth edition, New York: Macmillan, 1975.

Graedon, Joe, *The People's Pharmacy,* New York: St. Martin's Press, 1976.

Gulick, W. ed., *Consumer's Guide to Prescription Prices,* Syracuse: Consumer Age Press, 1973.

Hansteen, V. and E. Lorensten, "Vasodilator drugs in the treatment of peripheral arterial insufficiency," *Acta. Med. Scand.* [Suppl.], 556:3-62, 1974.

Heinonen, O.P. et al., "Reserpine use in relation to breast cancer," *Lancet,* 2(7882):675-77, 1974.

IMS America, (comp.), *National Disease and Therapeutic Index,* Ambler, PA, 1975.

—————————, *National Prescription Audit: Therapeutic Category Report,* Ambler, PA, 1979.

Kastrup, E.K., ed., *Facts and Comparisons,* St. Louis: Facts and Comparisons, Inc., August 1980.

Lee, G. et al., "Antianginal efficacy of oral therapy with isosorbide dinitrate capsules," *Chest,* 73:327-32, 1978.

Long, J.W., *The Essential Guide to Prescription Drugs,* New York: Harper & Row, 1977.

Melman, K.L., and H.F. Morelli, *Clinical Pharmacology,* New York: Macmillan, 1972.

Naide, D., "Vasodilators for arterial insufficiency," *American Family Physician,* 22(1):128-129, 1980.

North American Contact Dermatitis Group, "Epidemiology of Contact Dermatitis in North America: 1972," *Archives of Dermatology,* 108:537-40, 1973.

Page, L.B. et al., "Medical management of primary hypertension," *New England J. Med.,* 287:1018-1023, 1972.

Patrick, J., J.D. Panzer and V.J. Derbes, "Neomycin sensitivity in the normal (nonatopic) individual," *Archives of Dermatology*, 102:532-35, 1970.

Penna, R.P., ed., *Handbook of Nonprescription Drugs*, sixth edition, Washington: American Pharmaceutical Association, 1979.

Ronnov-Jessen, V. and A. Tjernlund, "Hepatotoxicity due to treatment with papaverine: report of four cases," *New England J. Med.*, 281:1333-35, 1969.

Silverman, H.M. and G.I. Simon, *The Pill Book*, New York: Bantam, 1979.

Stern, R.S., et al., "Risk of Cutaneous Carcinoma [skin cancer] in Patients Treated with Oral Mexthoxsalen Photochemotherapy for Psoriasis," *New England J. Med.*, 300:809-13, 1979.

Tomatis, L., "Carcinogenicity of phenacetin," *Science*, 204 (4389): 129-130, 1979.

"Vaginal sulfa agents should be banned, says FDA group," *Medical World News*, 20: 34-37, 1979.

Zetterquist, S., "Muscle and skin clearance of antipyrine from exercising ischemic legs before and after vasodilating trials," *Acta. Med. Scand.*, 183:487-496, 1968.

Zimmerman, H.J., "Papaverine revisited as a hepatotoxin," *New England J. Med.*, 281:1364-65, 1969.

These drugs are no longer being manufactured as of 1981 but will probably remain available for the next few years because some stores will still have stock manufactured before 1981.

Angitrate #10
Angitrate #20
Antora-B TD
Antora TD
Biozyme Ointment
Bromatapp Tablets
Butigetic
Butiserpazide Prestabs 25, 50
Carbrital Kapseals Half Strength
Cardilate P
Dainite
Dexamyl
Dialex 2.5
Dialex 6.5
Diphen-Ex Syrup
Eskatrol
Genespas-PB Elixir
Indogesic
K-Pava
Laserdil
Lobac
Luftodil
Naptrate Spancap
Neo-Corovas-30 Tymcaps
Neo-Corovas-80 Tymcaps
Neo-Polycin
Nitrine TDC

Nitro TD
Nitro-Lor
Nitrosule
Nitrovas
Nitrozem
Pava-2
Paveril Phosphate
PBZ Expectorant w/Ephedrine
    and Codeine
Pentraspan-30
Pentraspan-80
Pentryate Stronger
Perihab
Priscoline
Priscoline Lontabs
Rate-T-30
Reithritol
Sedralex
Sorbide-10
Spastyl
Spastyl w/Phenobarbital
Spentapp Tablets
Sulfathalidine
Tarcortin
Tri-Pavasule 300
Vasodil